THE ROOTS OF DISEASE

THE ROOTS OF DISEASE

CONNECTING DENTISTRY AND MEDICINE

ROBERT KULACZ, D.D.S.
AND THOMAS E. LEVY, M.D., J.D.

FORWARD BY JAMES EARL JONES

Copyright © 2002 by Robert Kulacz, D.D.S. and Thomas E. Levy, M.D..

Library of Congress Number:		2002090685
ISBN :	Hardcover	1-4010-4895-1
	Softcover	1-4010-4894-3

All rights reserved. No part of this book may be reproduced or transmitted in any form or by any means, electronic or mechanical, including photocopying, recording, or by any information storage and retrieval system, without permission in writing from the copyright owner.

This book was printed in the United States of America.

To order additional copies of this book, contact:
Xlibris Corporation
1-888-795-4274
www.Xlibris.com
Orders@Xlibris.com

CONTENTS

ACKNOWLEDGMENTS 9
INTRODUCTION 11
FOREWORD BY JAMES EARL JONES 15

**1 ROOT CANAL PROCEDURES:
    ANATOMICAL AND CLINICAL ASPECTS 19**
   None of the Usual Suspects 19
   What Isn't Taught Doesn't Exist 21
   Anatomy of the Root Canal 23
   Why a Root Canal Procedure is Performed 24
   The Exceptional Toxicity of an Abscessed Tooth 25
   Eliminating Pain While Preserving Infection 26
   Save the Tooth or the Body? 29
   Another Example 30
   A Historical Note 32

**2 DOCUMENTING THE TRUTH: THE
    RESEARCH OF DR. PRICE 34**
   A Distinguished Reseacher 34
   Focal Infection 35
   Focal Infection: Historical Roots 37
   Focal Infection: Dental Roots 38
   Scientific Literature Overview 38
   Are All Root Canal Treated Teeth Infected? 42
   Toxic Effects Without Bacteria 45
   Non-Toxic Effects of Uninfected Teeth 45
   Position Statement of the AAE on Focal Infection 46
   The Model of Toxic Shock Syndrome 47

3 MORE OFFICIAL POSITIONS 52
   The American Dental Association (ADA) 52
   The ADA and Root Canal Procedures 56
   A Slow Awakening: Personal Notes 58
   Claims and Counterclaims 60

4	**THE FOCUS IN DENTAL SCHOOL** **64**
	The Drive to Save Teeth 64
	Faking It to Graduate 66
	Guarding Your Territory 67

5	**IGNORING THE FACTS** **68**
	The Need for Comprehensive Treatment Plans 68
	Seven Important Questions About Root Canal Procedures 72
	Some Endodontist "Answers" 73

6	**THE DIRECT EVIDENCE** **76**
	Sterile Instruments, Infected Teeth 76
	Seeing and Smelling Is Believing 78
	Prevention Versus Prescription 79
	Life is a Many-Splendored Thing 80
	Variable Immune System Strength 82
	Conditions Favoring Toxicity 84
	Additional Concepts of Infection 87
	The Fatally Flawed Root Canal Procedure: An Unreachable Primary Goal 88
	Testing for Toxins 91
	Desperately Seeking Sterility 92

7	**HIDDEN GANGRENE: THE CAVITATION** **100**
	Overview 100
	Historical Perspectives 101
	Diagnosis 103
	X-Raying the Invisible? 105
	Physical Appearance and Characteristics 106
	New Technology 108
	Cavitation Frequency 109
	Treatment of Cavitations 111
	When the Batteries Die: A Case History 113
	Dental Implant Toxicity 118

8	**PROPER PRE-OPERATIVE AND POST-OPERATIVE CARE** **124**
	Overview 124
	Weighing Risk Versus Benefit 125

Oral Pathogens and Systemic Effects 126
Practical Prevention and Protection 127
Reducing Oral Microbes 128
Antibiotic Administration 129
Protecting the Gut 129
Other Protective Measures 130
Unipolar Magnetic Therapy 131
Summary 132

9   PERIODONTAL DISEASE 133
Overview 133
Clinical Consequences of Periodontal Disease 136
Treating and Preventing Periodontal Disease 139
Summary 140

10 FREQUENTLY ASKED QUESTIONS 141
What is a root canal procedure and why is it performed? 141
Does a root canal procedure remove all
of the infection from the tooth? 142
Isn't there anything that can be used
to sterilize the bacteria in these dentin tubules? 144
Why can't a laser sterilize the tubules? 144
I heard that there is a material called Biocalex that is supposed to
penetrate the dentin tubules and kill bacteria. Would this be an
option for effective sterilization of root canals? 145
What about ozone treatment? 146
Why not just take out the root canal and leave the tooth? 147
How do I know if this root canal treated tooth is affecting my
health? Will my physical ailments get better if I extract
root canal treated teeth and I have cavitations cleaned out? 147
What if I don't get better after the extraction of a root
canal treated tooth or after cavitation surgery? 148
Should antibiotics be used during extractions
and cavitation surgery? 149
How can the risk of infection
be reduced during oral surgery? 150
What should I do first: have my amalgams replaced or have my
root canal treated teeth extracted and my cavitations cleaned? 151
Is there any way to tell if my root canal is toxic? 151

11 PATIENT TESTIMONIALS 153

APPENDIX I
SURGICAL PROTOCOL FOR TOOTH
EXTRACTIONS AND CAVITATION SURGERY 175

APPENDIX II
SELECTED ABSTRACTS FROM
THE SCIENTIFIC LITERATURE 182
I. Articles Documenting the Associations Between
   Dental Microbes and Systemic Disease 183
II. Cavitation Articles 204
III. Articles on Dental Toxins 216
IV. Articles Examining Sources of Dental Infection 220
V. Articles Documenting the Chronic Infections in
   Root Canal Treated Teeth 223

APPENDIX III
CAUSES OF CAVITATIONS
AND ASSOCIATED CONDITIONS 234

APPENDIX IV
PHOTOGRAPHS 243

APPENDIX V
RESOURCES 256

APPENDIX VI
ABOUT THE AUTHORS 259

ACKNOWLEDGMENTS

Although there are two authors' names on this book, this book was actually due to the efforts of many individuals. Numerous individuals have influenced us, taught us, supported us, and mentored us. I [RK] would first like to thank my wife Susan, who, as a physician, mother, editor, and wife, has been a solid foundation for our family. Her love, companionship and support helped me pursue my academic curiosities.

My mother and father, Robert and Kathleen Kulacz, who always wanted the best for their children, sacrificed much to help me attain my education. They continue to help our family to this day as parents and as grandparents. I cannot thank them enough for their past and present support and love.

Dr. Larry Klotz, my professor and student advisor as an undergraduate student at S.U.N.Y., Cortland, and Dr. Herb Gross, one of my professors at New York University College of Dentistry deserve specific thanks. Both set examples of complete integrity in the pursuit of academic truth.

Christopher Hussar, D.O., D.D.S. has devoted his life to the treatment of the systemic ramifications of oral disease. Dr.

Hussar has been a leader in the field of cavitation surgery and I am proud to call him my friend and colleague.

To my staff, Faith Billington, Sandy Bourne, Geraldine Osborne, Carol Grazioli, I thank you for your confidence in me to never compromise my treatment principles.

My friends Frank Schutte, Dan Honig, and Steve Feller, who have never faltered in defining true friendship, thanks.

I also wish to thank Cristin Grenier for her assistance in preparing this manuscript.

In addition to Dr. Kulacz's acknowledgments, Dr. Levy would like to thank Hal Huggins, D.D.S., M.S. for first introducing him to the overwhelming significance of dental toxicity nearly nine years ago. I [TL] feel that the contribution of Dr. Huggins to the awareness of the essential and irrefutable link between dentistry and medicine needs to be properly realized by all who have and will benefit from this vital information.

INTRODUCTION

This book was written because it had to be written. From both the dental and medical perspectives, we have seen an epidemic of the most widespread proportions continue to widen rather than lessen. The hidden infections found in all root canal treated teeth continue to be arguably the most significant cause of many serious degenerative diseases, most notably cancer and heart disease. It is our opinion that the evidence clearly shows that many, if not most, significant diseases and medical conditions get their start in the dentist's chair. Some of the dental procedures commonly performed every day by practicing dentists certainly initiate many, and worsen most, medical conditions.

Root canal treated teeth are not the only sources of dental infection, although they are probably the most significant in terms of the severity of the diseases they cause. Cavitations are another major contributing source of dental toxicity that remains virtually unknown to the vast majority of practicing dentists today in both the United States and the rest of the world. The case histories that we have cited are nevertheless very real, and the number of people affected by the toxicity of cavitations exceeds even the number of people affected by the toxicity of root canal treated teeth. The vast majority of people who have ever had teeth extracted, especially the larger teeth such as the wisdom teeth and molars, are suffering from the toxicity of these gangrenous holes in their jawbones. This also means that older dental patients who may feel that they have "escaped" the many toxins associated with modern dental care when they finally get full-mouth extractions and dentures have only traded one form of dental toxicity for another form. The denture wearers uniformly have an enormous amount of cavitation-related toxicity. In isolated patients, cavitation toxicity can be as bad or worse than root canal treated teeth toxicity.

Another enormous source of infective dental toxicity that has gained publicity in the last decade or so is that of periodontal, or gum-related, disease. The association between variable degrees of periodontal disease and very significant medical diseases such as heart disease and stroke has received unequivocal confirmation in the medical and dental literature. It appears clear that any dental infection, whether it is gum-related, root canal-related, cavitation-related, abscess-related, or implant-related, has very consistent and serious medical consequences.

Much of what we have written about in this book relates to the concept of focal infection. A focal infection seeds microbes and their associated toxins throughout the body. The mouth continues to be the most significant source of these seedings. While we have attempted to relate a number of compelling case histories of patients we have encountered with dental toxicity and focal infection-related clinical syndromes, we have also included an extensive appendix at the end of this book. This appendix contains only a sampling of the very many pertinent abstracts from the current dental and medical articles in the scientific literature. The reader can choose to just read the bulk of this book and trust that we are relating scientifically valid observations, or the motivated reader can also find even greater definitive support for our position on the toxicity of dental infections from this appendix of cited abstracts.

The premises offered in this book do affect the financial livelihoods of a large percentage of dentists. While we don't intend to speculate on any theories of conspiracy or other such dark notions, it is very important to always fully appreciate the "money trail" when trying to understand why things work the way that they do. Presently, an endodontist who fully understood, appreciated, and *acknowledged* the validity of all the information presented in this book would simply have to stop doing root canal procedures. It is no surprise, then, that very few endodontists are open to even considering whether this information could be true. Ironically, if the discerning endodontist was reading this book carefully, it would be obvious to him or her that an enormous amount of work still remains to be done in order to properly address the untold numbers of cavitations that need proper surgical cleaning. Endodontists could very well end up becoming cavitation specialists after giving up doing root canal procedures. However, it would involve both a major change in dental practice, additional training, and a complete renouncement of the fatally flawed root canal procedure. Like most people, dental specialists such as endodontists don't like having the "rules" changed after their formal educations have been completed. Nor do they wish to entertain theories and concepts that conflict with the foundations of their original professional educations. Massive change will always be resisted, regardless of how appropriate that change may be. This is not to say that endodontists and other dentists intend to hurt anyone. They simply refuse to believe that a major change in the way they practice dentistry is in the best health interests of the public.

Unfortunately, the root canal procedure is presently being performed more frequently than ever before. By the early 1960's root canal procedures were performed in the United States at the rate of about 3 million per year. This rate increased to roughly 40 million per year by the early 1990's. Currently (2002) in the

United States more than 50 million root canal procedures are being performed per year. Since the international dental community largely follows the lead of the United States, the frequency of root canal procedures is similarly skyrocketing across the world. Even if modern medicine finds some way to keep patients alive while lessening their symptoms with prescription medications, chronic degenerative diseases can be expected to appear ever earlier in life as more and more root canal procedures are performed. Indeed, many cardiologists will tell you that only a few decades ago it was almost unheard of for a man in his 20's to sustain a heart attack. Now it is not so uncommon. We feel the evidence presented in this book clearly demonstrates that dental toxicity is a primary reason for the appearance of heart disease as well as many other chronic degenerative diseases.

From the perspectives of both dentistry and medicine, we believe the science supporting the toxicity of the root canal treated tooth, the cavitation, the implanted tooth, the abscessed tooth, and infected gum tissue is not in doubt, and actually has not been in doubt for a very long time. We feel very strongly that dentists and physicians must be guided entirely by what is scientifically true and by what is in the best health interests of their patients. The desire to avoid change and to regard all historical as well as current scientific beliefs as being beyond reproach and question must no longer play any role in health care. The education of our dentists and physicians must truly be a lifelong process that does not end upon acceptance of a diploma. The license to practice a dental or medical discipline is a privilege, not a right. Most education begins *after* the awarding of an academic degree. Dentists and physicians alike must take full responsibility for the welfare of their patients. They must always strive to attain the complete truth in their knowledge base, to follow the most effective of treatment philosophies, and to maintain the greatest of integrity in their care giving.

FOREWORD TO

THE ROOTS OF DISEASE:
CONNECTING DENTISTRY AND MEDICINE
BY ROBERT KULACZ, D.D.S.
AND THOMAS LEVY, M.D., J.D.

I took so much medicine I was sick a long time after I got well.
—Carl Sandburg, *The People, Yes*

I was fortunate to be raised in a household where folk medicine was common practice. Therefore, when I was growing up, *alternative* medicine was always an option. We lived on an isolated farm in Michigan back then, but my grandmother Maggie had grown up in rural Mississippi, attuned to folkways. My youngest uncle suffered from epilepsy in those days before there was any reliable treatment for controlling seizures. I remember how Maggie would hover over him when he had a seizure, dribbling a thimbleful of laundry bluing into his mouth.

That was the remedy she had learned in Mississippi. (To this day, probably out of dread, I have never identified the specific ingredient in the laundry bluing manufactured in the thirties that was supposed to help my uncle recover from his seizures. But the important thing was that Maggie believed the treatment worked, and because she believed it, my uncle did, too.)

Years later, because of an accident I had on a movie set, the cartilage in my knees had virtually given out. At one point I could barely walk. I was advised to go to New Mexico to try a therapy with a German doctor who was practicing holistic medicine. He gave me injections of bee venom in my knees and other pressure points, and my condition improved, at least to the extent that I could function again. I had been told that I would eventually need to have knee replacement surgery, but the idea was to forestall replacement as long as I could. My experience with bee venom was my first attempt to elect alternative means of healing.

Before I met Dr. Robert Kulacz, I needed root canal surgery. After a number of tests, it was determined I should be very careful about the kind of metal that went into my teeth. I set out to learn all I could about the risks of mercury fillings. At the time, more and more people were acknowledging the potential problems with mercury fillings, but most dentists were reluctant to consider alternate materials. They did not want to let go of traditional methods or established treatments. I wanted to find a dentist who was open to new procedures, and my search eventually led me to Bob Kulacz.

When I approached him, he was aware of the controversy about mercury fillings but he had not yet tried alternative treatments. Not only did Dr. Kulacz agree to give me fillings without mercury, his fascination with the whole subject led him into extensive research. As this book demonstrates, he opens his mind to new possibilities in his field, investigating and testing as he tries to find the best ways of caring for his patients.

The book Dr. Kulacz and Dr. Levy have written explores

the connection between dentistry and medicine. *Connection* is the key word here. Every human being is an entity of body, mind and spirit. In the universe of the human body, as the old song goes, "The head bone's connected to the neck bone," and so on. It is those dentists and physicians that look for connections who are most likely to serve their patients well. Not surprisingly, holistic medicine actively involves the patient as well as the doctor. The patient's obligation is to be as open minded and as aggressive as possible in the stewardship of his own health.

Laundry bluing, bee venom and an alternative to mercury: These three examples opened my mind. That is what I ask of you, the reader, as you pick up this book. Open your mind, and make your own thoughtful, informed decisions about what you may learn here.

—James Earl Jones

1

ROOT CANAL PROCEDURES: ANATOMICAL AND CLINICAL ASPECTS

None of the Usual Suspects

Mr. Smith's condition was deteriorating rapidly. It had been a month since his shortness of breath forced him to be admitted to the hospital. His family was gathered in a conference room along with two of his physicians. The pulmonologist, (lung specialist), spoke to the group:

> "We do not have any answers as to the cause of Mr. Smith's condition. We looked everywhere for a primary source for the infection but we found nothing."

At that point I [RK] felt compelled to speak up:

"No you didn't. You didn't check his mouth. Mr. Smith has two root canals and moderate to severe gum disease."

The pulmonologist appeared to completely ignore my comment, although his quick glance at the cardiologist sitting in the corner appeared to be an attempt to see if he had support in regarding me as another renegade dentist who just didn't get it. It was very clear to me that this doctor was not willing to even entertain the *possibility* of an oral focus as the cause of Mr. Smith's condition. Unfortunately, Mr. Smith died the next day.

With the family's permission I obtained Mr. Smith's complete hospital record. There were more question marks and frustrated uncertainties in the chart than there were definitive answers. It seemed that nobody had any idea why Mr. Smith was sick. Certainly, nobody put into writing any scientifically plausible hypothesis as to why Mr. Smith was so sick. Multiple consultations by a variety of medical specialists led to the same diagnostic dead end. Lacking any clear answers for his condition, these consultants literally flooded his body with antibiotics, even though all of the blood cultures testing for bacteria turned out negative. When the first set of antibiotics failed to produce any clinical improvement, different antibiotics were tried. This non-focused, machine gun-like administration of multiple drugs continued until Mr. Smith's kidneys and liver could no longer handle the toxic assault of the side effects of those drugs, along with the toxic effects of his underlying disease. Faced with this toxicity and the ongoing stress of the unchecked infection, these organs finally began to shut down. And, still, there was no diagnosis. There was never a diagnosis. The question marks continued to pile up in the medical record.

Mr. Smith, however, is not such an unusual case. Many people die every day in hospitals without a clear diagnosis. The final cause of death in such a patient commonly ends up being the "diagnosis," such as heart attack, blood clot, stroke, or respiratory failure. But what led up to so many of these "final causes" of death?

Sixteen years ago Mr. Smith had a root canal procedure on one of his teeth. During this treatment process he developed a heart infection known as subacute bacterial endocarditis (SBE). This infection was caused by bacteria from the infected tooth that had undergone a root canal procedure. These bacteria entered the bloodstream and traveled to Mr. Smith's heart, where the bacteria actually invaded and grew upon one of the heart valves. The damage to the heart valve was so severe that it became necessary to do a heart valve replacement surgery.

SBE is often a life-threatening illness. Although an infected tooth is not the only source of the bacteria or other microorganisms that can cause SBE, Mr. Smith's SBE was clearly traced to his root canal treated tooth. This raised a very significant and logical question: After already having had such a severe illness caused by a dental infection, why was the possibility of disease-provoking oral bacteria as a cause for Mr. Smith's *current* illness not explored? The answers will shock you. As we shall see, one or more root canal treated teeth should *always* at least be given consideration as a primary cause, or a secondary and contributory cause, in the vast majority of diseases and clinical syndromes.

What Isn't Taught Doesn't Exist

The dental school curriculum exposes students to the basic biological sciences, such as biochemistry and physiology. However, most students regard these courses only as necessary requirements for graduation. They are not viewed as important building blocks for achieving a comprehensive understanding of how the body works and how the diseases of the mouth affect the rest of the body. There are few references to general medicine in dental school training, and little, if any, practical integration of the basic sciences into the clinical practice of dentistry. The main focus of a dental education is on the clinical and technical skills necessary for the everyday practice of dentistry. The basic sciences that should be thoroughly understood by any person with the title of "Doctor" are almost completely neglected by students in the dental school curriculum. Most dentists graduating from dental school are lacking a true understanding of the basic sciences. Their knowledge of general medicine ends up being literally little more than that of laypersons, unless they are motivated to study medicine further on their own.

Similarly, physicians must also take the basic biological science courses in medical school. But they, too, end up primarily focused on the clinical and practical aspects of their educations. There is very little mention of dentistry in medical school. Physicians are not trained in the diagnosis or treatment of dental disease, and they certainly receive no education regarding the materials used in dentistry. It's almost as if there is an unspoken understanding between dentistry and medicine that one has nothing to do with the other! Therefore, it should come as no surprise that many medical diseases caused by dental infections often go undiagnosed. In fact, as we saw earlier, it is rare that a dental infection such as is found in the root canal treated tooth is even given consideration as a possible contributing cause to a medical condition.

So, herein lies the problem. Dentists are not trained in medicine, and physicians are not trained in dentistry. In other words, NOBODY IS MINDING THE STORE! Both the medical and dental professions have largely ignored the vital mutual relationship between their respective disciplines. However, we will see that this was not always the situation. But let us first try to understand better what a "root canal" is, which is the common way of referring to a root canal treated tooth. Then, we will see why this dental infection is so often devastating to the overall health of the patient.

Anatomy of the Root Canal

How can such a benign-appearing procedure as a root canal procedure cause serious medical problems? To answer this question we must first understand the anatomy of a tooth. After that, we will then see what a root canal procedure is and why it is performed.

A tooth is anchored in the jawbone by its root. A front tooth usually has one root, and a molar, a larger back tooth, can have as many as three or more roots. Each of the roots has a nerve supply and a blood vessel supply, which enter the bottom of the root from the jawbone. These nerves and blood vessels extend up the root into an area called the pulp chamber. From this inner pulp chamber, or main canal, there are also multiple minor canals that branch off. These are called lateral canals. These lateral canals extend outward to the periphery, or outside containment area, of the tooth root. The rest of the entire structure of the tooth between the outer enamel coating on the visible crown portion of the tooth and the thin covering of cementum encasing the buried root in the jawbone is composed of a substance called dentin. It is in this dentin that we find the main problem with root canal treated teeth.

Dentin is not a solid substance. It is richly porous, much like a sponge. This porous structure is composed of a fine network of microscopic channels called dentin tubules. These tubules are so numerous that if you were to place the tubules from even the smaller front tooth end-to-end they would stretch for three miles! And, as tiny as they are, they are still wide enough to easily accommodate bacteria and other infecting microbes. So, an infected tooth is capable of indefinitely harboring literally millions of bacteria or other microbes within its dentin tubules. Either trauma, deep decay, or the root canal procedure itself is the primary reason for the introduction of this infection into the tooth.

Why a Root Canal Procedure is Performed

When a cavity gets so large that the bacteria responsible for the decay finally invade and infect the pulp chamber, traditional dentistry will try to "save" the tooth by offering the patient a root canal procedure. Only after multiple root canal procedures have been performed on such a tooth and the patient's main symptom, usually pain, remains unrelieved, will extraction of the tooth be finally offered by the dentist to the patient.

Eventually this infection within the pulp chamber will cause the tissue within the canal space to die. Usually the infection will even extend past the apex (tip) of the root, causing destruction and further infection of some of the anchoring jawbone. A dentist can sometimes, but not always, see this destruction on an x-ray of the root. There is usually a moderate amount of pain associated with such an infection, but not always.

When a dentist performs a root canal procedure on an infected tooth, the infected nerves, blood vessels, and connective tissue are routed out of the pulp chamber and the main canal space as completely as possible. This primary canal is then shaped, widened, and finally filled with a rubber-like material called gutta percha, combined with a sealing material. The stated goal of this procedure, according to the American Association of Endodontists (AAE), is the elimination of bacteria within the tooth. The AAE is the organization of dentists who do most of the root canal procedures. Endodontists receive additional training after dental school graduation, and they are regarded as the specialists in performing the root canal procedure.

However, there is a major problem with achieving this goal of sterility. The lateral canals that we described earlier, which can harbor diseased tissue and bacteria, are not accessible by the standard root canal procedure, and they simply cannot be cleaned out. Similarly, there is no way to reach and eliminate the bacteria that are hiding in the dentin tubules, which is like having thousands more microscopic lateral canals. No amount of medications used to try and sterilize the dentin tubules has *ever* been shown to be completely effective. Nearly all of the teeth treated with a root canal procedure harbor bacteria from the moment the procedures are completed! Furthermore, bacteria will eventually migrate into, and be harbored by, the root canal treated tooth. This occurs regardless of how well the procedure is performed. This means that all root canal treated teeth are still infected or will soon become infected after the procedure is completed, even though the supposed goal of the procedure is to eliminate infection. In fact, many root canal procedures are performed primarily to eliminate or minimize *pain*, and this goal is typically accomplished while infection remains, since many of the nerves and nerve endings are literally removed from the inside of the tooth. But eliminating pain in a tooth by a root canal procedure is an entirely different issue from eliminating the bacteria and other microorganisms infecting that tooth.

The Exceptional Toxicity of an Abscessed Tooth

An even worse scenario for the immediate health of a patient occurs when an infected tooth with an abscess or cyst in the surrounding bone goes untreated. Such a tooth has abundant bacteria and necrotic (dead) material in the main pulp chamber. In contrast, a root canal treated tooth has had at least a portion of the infected and necrotic pulp chamber removed during the root canal procedure. This immediate reduction in the infectious load of a root canal treated tooth allows it to be less acutely toxic than a grossly abscessed tooth. Of course, the chronic toxicity of the root canal treated tooth remains unaffected. Nevertheless, it is important to realize that an abscessed tooth without treatment can be expected to be the most toxic tooth simply because it has the highest abundance, or quantity, of contained infection and associated toxins.

Eliminating Pain While Preserving Infection

What happens to the bacteria that are left trapped within the lateral canals and the many dentin tubules?

It would be nice to think that they are neatly locked inside the tooth, incapable of causing any harm. In fact, that is what many endodontists believe. They feel that since there are many areas of the body that are not completely sterile in the absence of illness, it is also not important that a root canal treated tooth be completely sterile after the procedure either. They presume that the patient's immune system will "handle" any of the bacteria or other microbes remaining in the evacuated root canal space. The problem with this concept is that some areas of the body are supposed to always remain sterile, unviolated, and never directly challenged by bacteria or other infectious agents. The tooth pulp is one of those areas.

Also, remember that there are good bacteria and there are even more pathogenic, or disease-causing, bacteria. The normal bacteria found in the intestine are "friendly" bacteria that are helpful to the body. These bacteria help prevent the growth of pathogenic bacteria and other microbe forms such as yeast. But sometimes "good" bacteria can *become* "bad" bacteria. Just like *Clostridium botulinum*, the species of bacteria that produces the extremely potent toxin associated with botulism, many bacteria normally found in the mouth are virtually harmless to the body until their oxygen supply is taken away. Once this occurs, the lack of oxygen changes the metabolism of the bacteria, and enormously toxic bacterial metabolic by-products are produced. Just as the botulism bacteria will produce botulism toxin in the oxygen-starved environment of a contaminated vacuum-packed can of food, the harmless bacteria of the mouth will produce similarly potent toxins when trapped in the oxygen-starved environment of the dentin tubules of a root canal treated tooth.

Any such tooth that has been infected by the presence of these bacteria will eventually contain some dead pulp tissue. This sometimes creates a pus-containing abscess at the tip of the root. However, once the anatomy of the tooth has been physically altered by the root canal procedure, there appears to be no way by which the immune system can restore and then maintain the necessary sterility of the tooth pulp, even if no frank abscess develops. In other words, the root canal procedure is a *fatally flawed procedure*. The very nature of the procedure itself prevents it from achieving its supposed primary goal: a non-infected, sterile tooth.

Why do most root canals seem to be clinically successful? A root canal is judged to be a success when the pain has gone away and the bone around the root that was previously involved with the infection *appears* healed on x-ray examination. Most endodontists will perform a root canal procedure on any tooth that is technically treatable by the procedure regardless of the degree of infection or of the virulence and disease-causing capabilities of the microbes that are involved. In fact, a grossly infected tooth is one of the primary reasons that many root canal procedures are performed! The endodontist actually persists in thinking that the root canal procedure can sometimes eliminate the infection in such a tooth.

I [RK] observed this first-hand when a physician in my town had a problem with a root canal treated tooth. This physician had a root canal procedure started on a front tooth on a Thursday. By Saturday he was in so much pain that he called his endodontist back. The endodontist agreed to see him that morning, and proceeded to drain the infection from the tooth and to irrigate the inside of the pulp chamber. Remember that an endodontist specializes in the technical ability to do or redo the root canal procedure. Extracting such an infected, painful tooth is diligently avoided, since extraction of the tooth is perceived by the endodontist as a sign of professional defeat and technical incompetance.

On his way home, the physician began to feel extremely ill. He told his wife to drive him to the hospital emergency room. Upon arrival he was barely lucid. He was running a high fever, his heart rate was above 160 beats per minute, and his blood pressure was dangerously low. He kept pleading with the emergency room staff not to let him die. The doctor was then admitted to the intensive care unit in a state of severe toxic shock. The infectious disease specialists began treating him with antibiotics. The antibiotics they chose were primarily useful in killing aerobic bacteria, which are bacteria that thrive in the presence of oxygen. However, they were much less effective against the bacteria inside the root canal treated tooth, since those bacteria were living in an oxygen-deprived environment. Furthermore, the routing out of the blood vessels in the pulp chamber made it effectively impossible to assure the delivery of significant amounts of antibiotics to the inside of the tooth where the infection persisted and originated. Therefore, the antibiotics administered were of relatively little use in fighting this infection. In addition, it was the toxins that the bacteria produced that were introduced into the blood stream just a few hours before, when the dentist was treating the root canal, that caused the toxic shock.

Antibiotics can only affect the bacteria directly. Antibiotics have no effect at all on the toxins that these bacteria have already produced. Neither the physicians nor the attending dentists were familiar with the oral bacteria and their pathogenicity in an oxygen-starved environment, resulting in the mismanagement of the patient. Fortunately, this particular patient was an otherwise healthy young man with a relatively strong immune system. He was released from the intensive care unit after three days of being extremely ill with no apparent permanent damage. Had he been older or more immunologically compromised the outcome would likely not have been so favorable. But younger and stronger immune systems will often make clinical mismanagement look like appropriate, or at least acceptable, care.

Save the Tooth or the Body?

It would now seem logical that you should have a tooth that nearly killed you extracted as soon as possible. In fact, that is what I recommended. However, I received a call from an oral surgeon on the hospital staff who felt that the tooth could be saved by another root canal procedure. He stated that we had to try and save this tooth since this physician was a prominent member of the medical staff and the community. The physician's primary dentist also felt that the tooth could, and should, be saved by another root canal procedure. In the face of these identical recommendations, then, the physician decided to have the root canal procedure performed again. As mentioned earlier, there are few endodontists who do not believe that all cosmetically restorable teeth are indefinite candidates for repeated root canal procedures.

Meanwhile, the same bacteria that nearly killed the physician earlier remain lurking in the porous dentin tubules of his root canal treated tooth. His next illness only awaits the eventual inability of his immune system to keep on fighting this chronic infection and to keep on neutralizing the potent bacterial toxins being chronically released. That failure of the immune system may take days, weeks, months, and sometimes years. Furthermore, this eventual immune failure will often present as a life-threatening disease, such as a heart attack, or even as the ultimate disease of immune failure, cancer. And when such a disease occurs years after the root canal procedure was performed, the appropriate correlation between this flawed procedure and the onset of the disease is rarely made. As a result, the root canal treated tooth remains in the jawbone, and the chronic infection and toxin production in that tooth continues. This is why so many diseases are never self-limited once they are contracted. Rather, the immune compromise from the infection and toxicity of the root canal treated tooth only favors progression of the disease, not regression or recovery.

Another Example

Elizabeth was a 33-year-old female of normal height and weight with no history of any significant medical problems. One day she began having pain in the right kidney area. Her symptoms escalated to bouts of vomiting and diarrhea. Elizabeth's blood pressure was severely elevated, she was rapidly losing weight, and she was suffering from extreme fatigue. Elizabeth's internist was concerned enough about her clinical appearance that she was then admitted to the hospital. Medications were given to control her blood pressure, and antibiotics were given to fight the apparent kidney infection. Although Elizabeth showed slight improvement while in the hospital, she still had pain in her right kidney area. She was also having difficulty keeping food down, and she continued to lose weight. Her doctors told her that it would take at least six months for her to get better and that there was nothing more that they could do. She was released from the hospital and was monitored as an outpatient.

Instead of getting better, Elizabeth began getting worse. Her family did not know what to do. The doctors did not seem to have an answer, and Elizabeth's health continued its rapid decline.

Elizabeth's mother heard from a relative about my work with infected teeth and their effect on general health. Although they had their doubts about how a tooth could cause such a serious medical condition they felt that they were at the end of the road, and no traditional medical options remained. Elizabeth and her family felt at this point that anything was worth a try.

When Elizabeth arrived in my office her general appearance was poor. She was extremely thin with a pale complexion, and she could barely walk into the treatment room without feeling exhausted. After a thorough medical history, I [RK] did a dental exam. The dental exam showed that Elizabeth had one infected root canal treated tooth and two other infected molars. Although she had *no pain* associated with these teeth, both the clinical exam and the x-ray exam confirmed the infection. It is always extremely important to evaluate all of the teeth under such circumstances, not just those that are painful. When the immune system has been chronically weakened by a root canal treated tooth, other infected teeth will sometimes not be clinically apparent. Remember that pain, inflammation, and pus production are indicators that the immune system is doing its job. Lack of these signs can just mean that the immune system needs to be unburdened, such as from the toxicity of a root canal treated tooth, before it can recover enough to react appropriately against other sub clinically infected teeth. Although not a frequent occurrence, removal of one or more root canal treated teeth can result in the seemingly "spontaneous" infection of other teeth several weeks or months down the road. Such teeth were really just normal-appearing teeth with low-grade infection against which the immune system was finally able to exert a normal immune response.

Elizabeth then had the relationship between infected teeth and the rest of the body explained to her. She was told that if she were to present to her physicians with an infection on her hand of the same severity as was present in her teeth that it would receive top priority as a possible cause of her medical condition. But because physicians are not trained to look for dental disease as a cause for disease elsewhere in the body they did not even consider this possibility. And, of course, most dentists feel that dental disease is confined to the mouth only. Once again, nobody was minding the store!

Although the importance of having the infected teeth removed was stressed, Elizabeth could not be guaranteed that they were causing her present condition. Another undiagnosed, non-dental infection could still be at least part of the reason for her illness. Nevertheless, Elizabeth elected to have the infected teeth removed.

Within days Elizabeth began to feel better. Two weeks after the extractions she went back to her physician. The physician found that Elizabeth's blood pressure had returned to normal, and the high blood pressure medication being administered to Elizabeth was discontinued. When Elizabeth explained to her doctor that she had three infected teeth removed and asked him if that could have been the source of her problem, he said that it was "only a coincidence" and that the extraction of the teeth had nothing to do with her improvement. Even when these dental reasons for diseases are literally staring some doctors and dentists in their faces, awareness of this critical and common link between medicine and dentistry rarely occurs.

Within one month Elizabeth gained back all of her weight plus five pounds more. She said she was feeling fantastic. Before the extraction of the infected teeth Elizabeth's health had continued to decline for months. After the extractions her health immediately improved. The connection between the mouth and the rest of the body was indisputable in Elizabeth's case. Yet, medical schools and dental schools still do not teach these important associations, so they remain unknown to most doctors and dentists for the entirety of their professional careers, and many other "Elizabeths" just slip through the cracks.

A Historical Note

In 1913, Charles Mayo, M.D. said the following:

> It falls upon the dentist and oral surgeon to study the diseased conditions of the mouth. The work is discouraging, but it must be kept up, as eventually it will have its effect.

The next great leap in medical progress in the line of preventive medicine should be made by the dentists. The question is will they do it?

The answer to this question so far has been a resounding "NO," and almost a century has passed since Dr. Mayo's challenge. The integration of the disciplines of medicine and dentistry is very long overdue. The mouth is as integral a part of the human body as any other area, organ, or tissue. To ignore this important relationship between dental disease and general medical disease will just result in many more question marks on patients' charts. Physicians will continue to puzzle over the causes of many different medical conditions. As a result, untold numbers of people will suffer needlessly, take many toxic medications, and often die much, much too soon.

2

DOCUMENTING THE TRUTH: THE RESEARCH OF DR. PRICE

A Distinguished Reseacher

A New Truth a New Sense
The acquisition of a new truth is like the acquisition of a new sense, which renders a man capable of perceiving and recognizing a large number of phenomena that are invisible and hidden from another, as they were from him originally.

With this quote by Lieberg, Dr. Weston Price began his book that compiled much of his voluminous research on the fundamentals of dental infections and their effects throughout the body. Published in 1923, Volume I was entitled *Dental Infections: Oral and Systemic* and Volume II was entitled *Dental Infections and the Degenerative Diseases*. Dr. Price's exhaustive work examined the unequivocal links between dental infections and systemic disease. He also never found a root canal treated tooth that wasn't infected and toxic. And he looked at a very large number of root canal treated teeth. As we continue to see today, to our knowledge all root canal treated teeth when properly examined have proven to be infected and toxic.

A brilliant researcher, Weston A. Price, D.D.S., M.S., F.A.C.D., was the Director of the Research Institute of the National Dental Association for over 14 years. Desiring that his work remain scientifically pure without any suggestion of a secondary motive, he refused any salary during his tenure as director. He published over 220 papers and three major books during his lifetime. Both the medical and dental communities held Dr. Price in high esteem during his lifetime. Even the American Dental Association (ADA), which now would contest many of the results produced by his meticulous research, honored him for his outstanding contributions to the art and science of dentistry. Only after Dr. Price died was his landmark research eventually summarily dismissed as outdated. It would appear that no research could possibly be officially endorsed that so clearly demonstrated the enormous toxicity of the root canal treated tooth.

Focal Infection

Dr. Price's volumes of research on the links between oral infection and systemic disease were based on the concept of focal infection. Focal infection is defined as a secondary infection initiated at another site in the body by bacteria or their toxic by-products that have traveled from a different focus of infection. Simply stated, an infection in one part of the body can spread bacteria or bacterial toxins to another part of the body, causing disease at the new tissue site. This concept is generally accepted in the practice of medicine, although it is limited to certain well-recognized models, such as dental infection causing subacute bacterial endocarditis (see Chapter 1) and infected tonsils causing acute rheumatic fever and acute rheumatic arthritis.

Dentistry, too, accepts the validity of a limited number of focal infection models. However, dentistry completely misses the overwhelming impact of the most toxic and most common of the focal infections: root canal treated teeth. The American Association of Endodontists (AAE) put out a patient brochure in 1994 entitled "Are your root canals making you sick? Absolutely not!" Recall that endodontists are the dental specialists who spend nearly all of their time performing root canal procedures on teeth. Would it be very likely that any professional group will embrace that which would largely eliminate the primary source of their income? Unlikely.

In its patient brochure, the AAE addresses whether it believes the root canal treated tooth is a source of focal infection. It asserts that root canal treated teeth are absolutely safe. It further asserts that it has been proven beyond a shadow of a doubt that root canal treated teeth cannot harm the patient. The AAE claims that the cleaning-out and filling-up of the pulp root system in the root canal procedure destroys the bacteria present in an infected tooth, assuring that the root canal treated tooth cannot be a source of infection to other parts of the body. Furthermore, the AAE goes on to assert that as the science of dentistry progressed, more sophisticated research showed that the focal infection concept and Dr. Price were both wrong. Don't be surprised if you cannot find any of this supposed research. It doesn't exist.

Science and medicine often have to deal with what most scientists would want to believe rather than with what objective research reveals. Some of the highlights of Dr. Price's research will be cited, and if you have a skeptical but *open* mind, do go back to the books published by Dr. Price, and you will be presented with the most meticulous and detailed of research. Dr. Price's studies match and even exceed the quality of most research performed today. Good research does not age into bad research. It stands on its own merits indefinitely.

As we explore the research of Dr. Price and others, you will see how the AAE is simply wrong in its assumptions and assertions about the clinical impact of root canal treated teeth. Whether the unwavering support of the AAE toward its featured procedure is based on a perception that genuine scientific validation exists or based on an interest in self-survival will be for you to decide. After all, practitioners of techniques of dubious scientific merit, such as root canal procedures, often do not hesitate to use those same techniques on family members and other loved ones. Self-delusion can sometimes progress to mammoth proportions.

Focal Infection: Historical Roots

Throughout the last century, men such as W.D. Miller, William Hunter, Weston Price and Edward Rosenow proposed and researched the concept of focal infection. Their research repeatedly concluded that oral microorganisms and their toxic metabolic by-products were involved in a wide variety of systemic diseases that were not always of obvious traditional infectious origin. Rosenow hypothesized that bacteria would migrate from a primary source, often the mouth, to a distant site in the body. He proposed that this often unsuspected spread of infection would then result in a variety of clinical diseases, depending upon the ability of the traveling microorganism to survive and grow better at those new, remote sites in the body.

This phenomenon came to be termed "elective localization," as Dr. Rosenow was able to subsequently demonstrate in a test tube that the same microorganism might have different levels of virulence under variable conditions supporting growth. Generally, bacteria seek out body tissues with a certain microenvironment, such as a particular oxygen concentration, that is especially favorable for their growth. This tissue microenvironment may be different from one person to the next, depending upon such factors as genetics and previous injury to the tissue involved. And because this microenvironment may vary from one person to another, different diseases resulting from microbe localization in different tissues can develop in different people, even though the initial infecting microorganism is the same.

Focal Infection: Dental Roots

It is a well known and medically accepted fact that a variety of clinical dental procedures, including the extraction of a tooth, the performance of a root canal procedure, and the cleaning of infected gums, may cause the seeding of microorganisms from the oral cavity into the bloodstream. Ideally, microorganisms that gain access into the bloodstream from the oral cavity should be eliminated from the body within minutes by the immune system. However, in patients with diseases or conditions such as artificial heart valves, degenerating organs, vascular diseases, or artificial joints, blood-borne bacteria can pose a grave threat to health if the immune system cannot prevent them from taking hold and multiplying at these different sites. Patients who are immunocompromised, such as many older patients, patients with autoimmune diseases, or patients who have received long term steroid use, chemotherapy, radiation therapy, or immune system suppressing therapy (as in transplant patients), are even more susceptible. This is because their immune systems have become weakened and are not as capable of adequately destroying the bacteria.

Scientific Literature Overview

A review of the conclusions from the scientific literature over just the last twenty years verifies the important role of oral infection and oral pathogens as the cause of many different types of systemic diseases and complications. The significance of focal infection originating in the mouth has actually been documented in scientific literature going back centuries. Consider the following:

Head and Neck:

Direct oral infection has been clearly shown to spread from defined oral foci to various locations in the head and neck and to the mediastinum (chest area). Although relatively rare, many of these conditions are fatal. More common are conditions such as maxillary sinusitis and other infections of the superficial and deep facial tissues. Infection may spread to surrounding soft tissues, as in cellulitis, or it may involve the floor of the mouth or ethmoid areas. It can also cause a very serious condition known as cavernous sinus thrombosis.

Fascial Planes:

Fascial planes refer to the contact areas between adjacent tissues, often deeply situated, in the body. Infection spreading through the fascial planes nearest the teeth may lead to serious infections known as parapharyngeal cellulitis, retropharyngeal space infection, descending cervical cellulitis, mediastinitus, thoracic empyema, necrotizing fascitis, and pericarditis.

Eye:

Orbital space infection, superior orbital fissure syndrome, proptosis, subconjunctival ecchymosis, ptosis, ophthalmoplegia, pupil dilation, and interference with light reflexes have all been reported as resulting from dental infections. Dental infections may also play a role in other inflammatory eye conditions, such as uveitis and endophthalmitis. The close physical proximity of the eyes and the oral cavity appears to play an important role in these disease associations. Probably many known eye conditions can be at least partially caused or worsened by a dental infection.

Brain Abscesses:

In several cases, the contents from brain abscesses and dental lesions have been found to have the same pathogens. In some cases, the individuals have died in spite of vigorous treatment. In other cases, however, when the dental lesions were removed the brain abscesses diminished in size and the individuals returned to a state of good health. In one case where a patient experienced seizures and a progressive deterioration of mental and muscular competence due to a brain abscess, the patient's neurological function returned to normal after an infected tooth was removed.

Meningitis and Osteomyelitis:

Acute hemiplegia resulting from a dental abscess and paraplegia resulting from a metastatic paraspinal abscess following a dental extraction have been documented as occurring from associated focal infections, as have both meningitis and vertebral osteomyelitis.

Respiratory System:

In the respiratory tract, solitary lung abscesses have been traced back to dental infections. Of particular concern in the susceptible elderly population is aspiration pneumonia of oral microbial origin.

Cardiovascular System:

Infective endocarditis is the most definitive and well-documented example of focal infection, and both aerobic and anaerobic bacteria have caused it. Many patients who have experienced infective endocarditis had no prior knowledge of heart valve damage, which is often a predisposing factor in acquiring this infection. It is important to note that bacteremia, although seen more often after dental extractions, may also result from routine dental procedures such as interligamental injection, rubber dam placement, and cleaning of the teeth. Septicemia has also been reported as resulting from oral infections.

More recently, the research has indicated a strong link between infected gums and coronary artery disease leading to heart attacks (also see Chapter 9). A similar connection has also been made between dental infection and strokes. It is also likely that bacterial effects cause an increase in the release of inflammatory mediators known as cytokines that can help promote atherosclerosis, the disease process that gradually narrows and eventually blocks off blood flow in arteries. The effects of these cytokines are in addition to the more direct damage of the bacteria and their toxic by-products to the lining of the blood vessel walls. The bacteria commonly found in the mouth can cause an aggregation (clumping) of platelets, which can also lead to the blocking of an artery that can result in heart attack or stroke.

Gastrointestinal Tract:

Oral microbes have been implicated in the cause of inflammatory bowel disease, liver infections, gastritis, and both gastric and duodenal ulcers.

Fertilization – Pregnancy – Birth Weight:

Many other health care specialties are now considering the possibility of focal infection as a causative factor or contributing factor to the development of their particular disease processes. There are reports of dental infection being related to bacteria in the semen, with the bacteria found in the mouth samples being similar to the bacteria found in the semen. Interestingly, appropriate dental treatment also resulted in a clearing of the bacteria from the semen and restoring fertility. Animal research has also shown that infection with gram-negative, periodontitis-associated organisms may adversely affect pregnancy outcome. Furthermore, severe maternal inflammatory periodontal disease (in humans) is associated with an increased risk for miscarriage, low birth weight babies and pre-term labor.

Miscellaneous:
Chronic uticaria (hives), tetanus, gangrene of the tongue, and fever of unknown origin have all been found to result from focal infections originating from the relocation of oral microbes.

Are All Root Canal Treated Teeth Infected?

In a word, yes. Dr. Price suspected that root canal treated teeth would remain infected even after the most diligent and meticulously performed of root canal procedures. He was able to demonstrate that the bacteria left in the tooth or their toxic products could migrate out of the tooth and travel to other parts of the body. Remember that the tooth has lateral canals off of the primary pulp chamber, along with a porous network of dentin tubules that can harbor millions of microorganisms. Root canal procedures have never eliminated these bacteria and simply cannot eliminate them. In fact, Dr. Price found that it was extremely difficult to sterilize root canal treated teeth even after they had already been *extracted*! The high heat and harsh chemicals that he used for this sterilization could *never* be used in the mouth, yet endodontists persist in thinking that the mere flushing out and subsequent packing of the pulp chamber will somehow magically reach and sterilize the full extent of the miles of dentin tubules extending away from the pulp chamber.

Dr. Price performed many experiments that very elegantly demonstrated that both bacteria and their associated toxins can escape from a root canal treated tooth and that generalized, systemic diseases would result. He made numerous clinical observations demonstrating the resolution of a wide variety of medical conditions, ranging from rheumatoid arthritis to psychiatric disorders, following the extraction of root canal treated teeth. In several of his experiments, he surgically implanted extracted root canal treated teeth under the skin of rabbits. Dr. Price found that if the rabbits did not die first from the overwhelming toxicity of the implanted teeth, they often developed the same diseases that plagued the humans from whom the teeth were extracted. He repeated these experiments over and over and continued to obtain the same results.

As an example of his persistence in demonstrating the reproducibility of his work, Dr. Price extracted a root canal treated tooth from a patient suffering from a severe disease involving the central nervous system. This tooth was placed under the skins of 31 consecutive rabbits. *All* of the rabbits died, most of them within four days. Furthermore, *all* of the rabbits developed similar neurological symptoms as the patient from whom the tooth was initially extracted! Dr. Price would repeatedly verify not only the enormous toxicity of these extracted root canal treated teeth, he also demonstrated that there existed an uncanny specificity of these teeth to reproduce the different diseases of their human donors in their rabbit recipients. For example, if a patient presented with a kidney infection that resolved after extraction of a root canal treated tooth, and this tooth was implanted under the skin of a rabbit, the rabbit would develop the same kidney infection. Dr. Price found that various bacteria had an affinity for specific body tissues and would tend to migrate there. This is the phenomenon called elective localization, a term coined by its discoverer, Dr. Edward Rosenow, and discussed earlier.

Although the bacteria and toxins from root canal treated and other infected teeth can affect any organ, Dr. Price found that the heart and circulatory system were very commonly affected. One patient, a 49-year-old man who was experiencing pain in his chest, was diagnosed as having myocarditis (inflammation of the heart). This patient was found to have two infected molars. Anaerobic cultures made from these teeth were injected into two rabbits. One rabbit died in twelve hours and the second rabbit's heart became large and flabby. A large, flabby heart is often the result of a rapidly progressive myocarditis. It would appear that the cultures from these extracted teeth reproduced the heart disease seen in the man who had the infected teeth. Upon removal of these infected teeth all of this patient's symptoms improved.

This was not an isolated case. Dr. Price demonstrated dramatic improvement in numerous cases of systemic disease following the removal of root canal treated teeth, as well as the subsequent transmission of those same diseases into rabbits either from implantation of the root canal treated teeth under the skin or from injections of extracts from those teeth. His experimental technique was impeccable, and his results would be difficult to challenge by any reputable, objective scientist reviewing his work.

Still, root canal specialists today assert that Dr. Price's work is invalid and outdated. Furthermore, they regard any dentist ascribing to this focal infection concept and extracting "clinically restorable" teeth as practicing below the general standard of accepted dental care. They still don't realize or they just refuse to accept that a root canal procedure will *never* sterilize a tooth. In fact, the root canal procedure will eventually result in the infection of a tooth that was not already infected beforehand!

Toxic Effects Without Bacteria

Dr. Price was interested in determining if it was the bacteria only or possibly other products from root canal treated teeth that caused disease. He demonstrated that if the extracted root canal treated tooth was ground up and all the bacteria were filtered out, leaving just the soluble extract, an even *more* profound toxic effect was often achieved when this bacteria-free extract was injected into the rabbits. The rabbits would often get sick or die *sooner* than when they were exposed to the skin implantation of the entire tooth that still contained live bacteria! What Dr. Price was trying to show was that it may not be the actual bacteria that always caused disease, but in fact the enormously potent toxins that the bacteria produced. He theorized that by injecting only the toxins that the bacteria produced without the bacteria themselves, the immune system did not have a "head start" in mounting a defense against the infection. The presence of the bacteria seemed to "prime" the immune system to fight the assault from the toxins. Without the prior exposure to the bacteria, the potent toxins rapidly overcame the immune system and illness or death occurred more quickly.

Non-Toxic Effects of Uninfected Teeth

Dr. Price implanted uninfected extracted teeth under the skin or muscle of a rabbit to see what would happen. He also implanted sterilized objects such as coins to see if just the presence of a foreign body might cause disease. In all such implants nothing of consequence happened to the rabbits. The implanted objects, either uninfected teeth or other foreign bodies, ended up being encapsulated in a cyst-like sack, remaining sterile. All of the rabbits remained healthy. Clearly, it was something from the infected teeth that caused disease, not merely the presence of a foreign body under the skin.

Position Statement of the AAE on Focal Infection

The AAE publishes informational newsletters for the dental community several times a year. The 1994 Fall/Winter newsletter addressed the topic of focal infection. On the front-page in large letters it reads: "Root canal therapy safe and effective." The subsequent text asserts that extensive and meticulous investigations proved that root canal therapy is a safe and effective means for saving teeth and that root canal treated teeth do not serve as foci, or sources, for infection in other parts of the body. The AAE goes on to say in this newsletter that when an infection does spread from a root canal treated tooth, it only spreads to immediately adjacent structures and does not spread to other parts of the body. The AAE completely denies that bacteria or their associated toxins can spread to other parts of the body and cause disease.

This is an interesting assertion since the AAE has published a position statement regarding the use of a material called Sargenti paste that contains paraformaldehyde, which the AAE considers ineffective and unsafe. The reason that the AAE considers Sargenti paste unsafe is that the chemicals in the paste can leak out of the tooth and cause damage to the surrounding tissues. But, more importantly, the AAE states that scientific evidence has shown that these chemicals are *not* necessarily confined to the tissues near the root canal treated tooth! Instead, the chemicals in Sargenti paste have been found to travel throughout the body and have been shown to infiltrate the blood, lymph nodes, adrenal glands, spleen, liver, and brain. If these chemicals can travel from a root canal treated tooth to other parts of the body, *then so can bacteria and the chemical toxins that these bacteria produce*. Dissemination throughout the body of toxic dental chemicals is not somehow magically limited to just those materials. Any other toxins given a similar access to the body will also find their way to remote body tissues. If dentist-placed chemical toxins are found in distant body tissues, then bacterial toxins, which are bacteria-produced chemicals, must also be able to travel there. This follows from basic scientific logic. The body does not care where the toxin came from in choosing where it should be spread.

The Model of Toxic Shock Syndrome

Toxic shock syndrome is a disease first described in the late 1970's that was initially almost exclusively associated with women who used "super absorbent" tampons. The case fatality rate, or death rate, for tampon-induced toxic shock syndrome is about 6 percent. Experts estimate that only 10 percent of all cases are recorded. Therefore, it would appear that many cases of toxic shock syndrome go undiagnosed.

Toxic shock syndrome is caused by the *Staphylococcus aureus* species of bacteria. *S. aureus* is a bacterium that is capable of producing a very potent exotoxin called TSST-1. An exotoxin is a protein that is produced and secreted by certain bacteria, often only under certain environmental conditions such as is seen with oxygen deprivation. When these toxins are released in the human body they are capable of producing disease, and they can be expected to do so when enough toxicity is released. In *Cecil Textbook of Medicine,* 19th edition, the clinical presentation of toxic shock syndrome is described as follows:

> The patient, almost always unaware of the focus of toxin production, experiences the abrupt onset of high fever, myalgias (muscle pain), and profuse nausea, vomiting, and watery diarrhea. . . . The patient often becomes progressively more ill and is frequently in frank shock when presenting for care. A diffuse capillary leak syndrome rapidly develops, and the serum albumin concentration drops to less than 2 grams per ml. Hypotension and frank shock are common and are often associated with adult respiratory distress syndrome (ARDS), acute renal (kidney) failure, and abnormalities in

literally every organ system evaluated. For example, an altered state of mentation, hepatocellular (liver) malfunction, elevated levels of muscle enzymes, and thrombocytopenia (disruption of platelets). Antibiotics are useless since it is the exotoxin that the bacteria produce that does the damage, and not the bacteria themselves. In fact, bacteria can rarely be cultured from the patient's blood. Treatment is supportive along with removal of the foci of infection, in this case the tampon.

Toxic shock syndrome develops when the *S. aureus* bacteria invade the tampon and begin to multiply there. If the tampon is left in place for too long a period of time, the bacteria can multiply in great numbers. These bacteria then produce the TSST-1 toxin that leaks out of the tampon, eventually entering the bloodstream and traveling throughout the body. This toxin is so potent that a very small amount can be lethal.

Why can't the body kill these toxin-producing bacteria before they cause disease? The reason is that a tampon has no blood supply since it is not part of the body. Therefore, the white blood cells used by our body to fight infection cannot gain access to the bacteria in the tampon. However, the bacteria that grow in the tampon can get inside the tampon because it is a porous substance. There they can multiply and thrive since fluids, including old blood, can seep in and provide nourishment. The bacteria can continue to grow untouched by the immune system in a warm, moist, dark, bacteria-friendly environment until they produce toxins that can eventually spread to the rest of the body and cause a life-threatening illness. Toxic shock syndrome is a perfect model of a focal infection, that is, a bacterial focus at one site in the body subsequently causing disease in one or more distant sites. In the case of toxic shock syndrome, it would appear that the dissemination of the bacterial toxins and not the bacteria themselves is the primary reason for the development of the disease.

Although toxic shock syndrome can produce dramatic

harmful effects at numerous distant sites in the body, the actual focus of toxin production remains, officially, somewhat poorly defined. Again referring to *Cecil's Textbook of Medicine,* toxic shock syndrome is almost certainly caused by the production of one or more toxins at the site of a localized and often relatively asymptomatic or unnoticed infection with any strain of *S. aureus* capable of toxin production. This last statement is critical in understanding how a similarly "asymptomatic" root canal treated tooth can actually be highly toxic.

As was described earlier, a root canal procedure is almost always performed when the normally sterile pulp canal becomes infected with bacteria and then becomes painful. These bacteria invade the pulp and migrate down the root canal space and into the porous tooth structure composed of countless dentin tubules. There, just like with a tampon, the bacteria continue to grow in the warm, moist, dark, and now bacteria-friendly environment.

The reason the tooth becomes a bacteria-friendly environment after a root canal procedure is performed is because there is no longer a normal blood supply into and out of the tooth. Moreover, just like with the tampon model, the bacteria infecting the tooth are now effectively out of reach of the body's immune system. Antibiotics are also of little help since there is no blood supply to effectively deliver them to the infection. Therefore, these bacteria, up to 400 different species, continue to multiply and adapt to the lack of oxygen present in the tooth pulp, becoming vastly more toxic in the process. Interestingly, fungi and viruses have also been isolated from root canal treated teeth and, likewise, there is no way for the body's defenses to fight these invaders either. The tooth becomes a reservoir for pathogenic (disease-causing) microorganisms and the potent toxins these microorganisms produce. When they are present for long enough, the appearance of some kind of disease is largely inevitable.

Selecting cotton tampons and changing them frequently

can significantly reduce the risk of developing toxic shock syndrome associated with tampons. The problem with a root canal treated tooth is that it is an integral part of your body and cannot be "changed frequently." The infected tooth is a permanent focus of infection that has the potential to cause disease throughout the body for as long as it remains. Although the predominant bacteria in infected teeth are streptococci and not the staphylococci seen in toxic shock syndrome, streptococci are also capable of producing very potent toxins when deprived of oxygen, causing a streptococcal type of "chronic" toxic shock. Such a situation can eventually manifest as any of a multitude of different diseases, depending upon the genetic predispositions or "weaknesses" of the affected patients.

To recap, the similarities between root canal treated teeth and the "infected" tampons of toxic shock syndrome are as follows:

1. Both are full of bacteria.
2. Both have little or no oxygen present at their cores.
3. Both present a warm, moist, dark, bacteria-friendly environment.
4. Both offer a safe haven for bacterial growth, largely free from attack by the body's immune system and free from reliable access by antibiotics.
5. Both can cause disease in other parts of the body once enough bacterial toxins, and to a lesser extent the bacteria themselves, are released and disseminated.

The comparison between a root canal treated tooth and a tampon is useful in illustrating the mechanism of initial infection with subsequent dissemination of bacteria and bacterial toxins from that focus of infection. The clinical presentation of symptoms from a root canal treated tooth can vary from the acute onset of severe body-wide symptoms to the gradual presentation and development of delayed health problems that may not manifest themselves for many years.

3

MORE OFFICIAL POSITIONS

The American Dental Association (ADA)

Dentistry is threatening the very health of the public that trusts the profession to thoroughly research the procedures and products used in dental treatments. Every person seeking dental care should expect the dentist to use the safest dental materials and to fully understand and explain the potential risks of different treatment procedures. A sound treatment plan for dental care should incorporate the broad base of both current as well as past research knowledge. The emphasis of care should be on the health and well being of the patient, and not on the potential profit margin. Dentists must remember that their discipline is a health profession that deals with diseases of the oral cavity *and with the relationship between oral health and overall health*. Too many dentists have forgotten that the mouth is an integral part of the human body. Or perhaps this realization simply never hit home in the first place, since it is not part of the formal dental curriculum.

Procedures performed in dentistry can and do affect the entire body. We must begin to objectively look at the validity of the scientific reasons behind the procedures performed every day in dental offices, as well as the systemic effects that these procedures can have on the health of the individual. It would appear that for far too long the ADA has perpetuated what has turned out to be flawed science, seemingly ignoring sound scientific evidence in the interest of maintaining the status quo. As an example of this kind of activity, let us look at the ADA position on one of the most common procedures performed in the dental office: the placement of mercury-containing amalgam fillings.

The mercury in a dental amalgam filling, which comprises typically about 50% of the filling components, is a prime example of the lack of scientific objectivity practiced by the ADA. The ADA proclaims and asserts without the slightest hesitation or qualification that amalgam is completely safe as a dental restorative material. In fact, mercury is, and remains, the most toxic non-radioactive heavy metal known to man. The ADA originally stated that no mercury was released from amalgam fillings and that once mercury was combined with the other metals such as silver it became a stable compound and "biologically inert." "Biologically inert" means that there can be no significant interaction with, or negative health effects from, exposure to that substance. A stable compound should maintain its original composition, never releasing any of its components into the body.

Amalgam completely fails to meet these criteria for a stable, biologically inert compound. The ADA statements regarding these alleged properties of amalgam were completely refuted by scientific research published in the mainstream dental literature throughout the world. Specifically, dental amalgam is only a mixture, not a true alloy. A true alloy is heated and then cooled to form a homogeneous and stable compound, with the different components ending up being chemically bound to each other. Amalgam, however, is made by the dentist in the dental operatory by cold-mixing mercury with other metals such as silver, tin, copper, and zinc. The resultant mixture is neither chemically stable nor biologically inert. Mercury vapor can be shown to come out of this mixture, and any mechanical stimulation of the amalgam, such as occurs with chewing, will cause an accelerated release of mercury vapor. In addition, since mercury vaporizes at a relatively low temperature, hot foods and drink will further increase the rate of release of mercury from the fillings. And remember that all of these factors just *accelerate* the release of mercury from the amalgam. It has already been demonstrated scientifically and published in the literature that mercury vapor is released continuously from amalgam with no additional stimulating factors. With this knowledge alone it would seem that the mouth would be a very poor place to insert mercury!

Even the government has published its own data quantifying the amount of mercury vapor that escapes continuously from amalgam fillings. The United States Environmental Protection Agency (EPA), in a report to Congress in December of 1997, stated that the highest body burden of inorganic mercury comes from the release of this heavy metal from dental amalgam fillings. The report shows that the amount of mercury exposure from dental amalgams totals more than from any other sources, including food (such as fish and other seafood) and water. The EPA estimates of systemically absorbed mercury from dental amalgam were the same as those reported by the World Health Organization (WHO) and by medical textbooks such as *Goodman and Gillman's: The Pharmacological Basis of Therapeutics*. These estimates were *significantly higher* than mercury absorption estimates conceded to by the ADA. And remember that these ADA estimates only appeared after the ADA was confronted with the irrefutable scientific studies documenting that any mercury came out of the amalgam at all.

Amalgam use has been totally banned in Sweden and there

are severe restrictions on its use imposed by other countries. The WHO has asserted that there is *no* safe level for mercury exposure. Here in the United States leftover scrap amalgam must be stored in an airtight container and disposed of as hazardous waste! How can the same material be hazardous waste outside the mouth and be perfectly safe when it is placed in teeth and expected to stay there not for moments, but for years? Why is amalgam (which, incidentally, is *not* FDA-approved for safety) still used by the majority of practicing dentists? And why would the ADA fight so fiercely to proclaim mercury amalgam fillings as safe? Let's examine some possibilities.

One fact is that amalgam is cheap and easy to use. A dentist can place several amalgam restorations in the same amount of time that it would take to place a single non-mercury containing composite filling. Composite fillings are tooth-colored fillings that are bonded to the tooth. They are very technique-sensitive and require a great deal of skill to place. Many dentists are unwilling or just unable to learn the techniques required to properly place composite fillings. They may also feel that they cannot charge a high enough fee to cover the increased treatment time. In addition, insurance companies often do not pay for the placement of composite fillings in back teeth. And finally, all American dental schools continue to routinely train their students to just be mercury amalgam-placers. So, for most practicing dentists, amalgam remains the main restorative dental material, largely due to the unrelenting endorsement by the ADA that amalgam is completely safe.

One likely reason that the ADA continues to proclaim the safety of amalgam is that of legal liability. If the ADA ever admitted that the mercury in amalgam could cause physical harm, then the number of lawsuits against the ADA and practicing dentists by people with amalgam fillings would be staggering. The confidence in the dental profession would be eroded to a level of complete distrust. The insurance companies would lose billions of dollars in claims not only for the replacement of amalgam fillings but also from the probable increase in disability claims due to physical harm caused by mercury toxicity. The resultant economic cascade would make the tobacco company and asbestos lawsuits pale in comparison.

So, it would seem, the ADA does the only thing it feels that it can do: continue to assert that in spite of all the studies documenting the release of mercury from amalgams, amalgam is still a clinically safe filling material. It would also seem that the ADA is quietly hoping that newer materials will gradually replace amalgam as a filling material, and the whole mercury amalgam issue will then just go away. This would enable the ADA to avoid ever facing an acknowledgment that it supported the use of such a toxic material as dental amalgam. The ADA could say that amalgam was the best material at the time, without even having to address the issue of toxicity, and then assert that mechanically superior materials are now available and should be used in the future.

The ADA and Root Canal Procedures

A visit to the dentist is an anxiety-producing experience for many people. Dentists often hear their patients state that they would rather be any place other than in the dental chair. Fear of pain during and after dental procedures, the invasion of one's personal space, and even the fear of choking are but a few of the factors that contribute to dental anxiety. However, most patients cling to the belief that their dentists are highly skilled and educated, and that they are fully informed on the safety of the dental materials used and the procedures performed. Surely, the patient typically thinks, the ADA is continuously researching the safety of materials and informing the dentists and the public of its findings. Dentists should, as do all legitimate scientists, evaluate research data in an objective, unbiased manner. The integration of new information into treatment protocols should evolve without prejudice. Unfortunately, this does not appear to be occurring with any regularity within the dental profession.

Critical information about the toxicity of dental materials such as mercury amalgam and of dental treatments such as fluoridation and root canal procedures has yet to effectively reach either the public or even the treating dentists. Furthermore, these uninformed dentists tend to remain uninterested in any scientific research that contradicts what they have already learned. As Einstein said: "Few people are capable of expressing with equanimity opinions which differ from the prejudices of their social environment. Most people are incapable of such opinion." Such is the current state of the dental profession. Too many dentists appear to be unwilling to think on their own. They simply follow blindly what the ADA dictates as the current and expected standard of care. Unfortunately, this standard of care is often based on inaccurate, misleading, and sometimes simply false information when compared to what are now known to be scientifically documented facts. Failure to integrate scientific research from the world literature into clinical practice has occurred and continues to occur routinely. The dental profession vigorously upholds the status quo on the use of materials and procedures with seeming disregard for the health consequences that these decisions can have on the public. Unless one of a very limited number of journals, mostly from the United States, support a new treatment or question an old one, no significant changes seem to occur in American dentistry.

It is high time that the public knows the truth about the possible negative health effects of dental treatments. Physicians are not trained to look at dental diseases as they look at medical diseases and dentists have focused their attention on specific dental procedures with little or no emphasis on how these procedures might affect the rest of the body. As a result many dentists have become "tooth carpenters," or technicians just trained to fix things, priding themselves primarily on their mechanical abilities, rather than priding themselves as doctors treating the mouth as it relates to the whole body.

So the questions remain: Who, if anyone, is examining the important relationship between dental health and overall systemic health? Who is reviewing the literature to see if what the ADA, or anyone else, says is true or not? How can you be sure that the dentistry in your mouth is not causing disease somewhere else in your body? The answer to all of these questions is that currently in the United States, the government, the public and the dentists remain unenlightened and seemingly even mislead by the ADA about the negative health effects of dental products such as mercury amalgam and fluoride. Similarly, neither the dentists nor the bulk of the public ever learn of the enormous toxicity that results from the root canal procedure. And if the ADA itself does not really know about these negative effects of dentistry on health, this is equally unacceptable. As a result of this lack of knowledge, neither your physician nor your dentist is likely to have any significant understanding of the complex relationship between oral health and systemic disease. This book can help you to become an educated dental consumer, and it will reveal to you some of the inexcusable and perhaps even negligent practices occurring regularly in the dental profession.

A Slow Awakening: Personal Notes

The manifestations of mercury vapor toxicity happened to me [RK] very slowly. At the time, I was placing and removing a large number of mercury amalgam fillings. At first, I would get frequent headaches while at work in my dental practice. Gradually, I noticed the presence of what I could only describe as "brain fog." This brain fog manifested itself as a decreased ability to think clearly, coherently, and at times as an inability to converse without losing my train of thought. I found it difficult at times to put thoughts together during a conversation.

Then I began feeling a tingling in my left hand along with a mild lessening of my coordination. Although nobody else could notice these subtle changes, I knew that something was not right. These symptoms would subside slightly during my days off work and would lessen even more during extended vacations, only to promptly return after I resumed my dental practice. Then came the most distressing symptoms of all. I began having brief periods of what I now acknowledge was mild depression and anxiety for seemingly no reason at all. Suddenly, the little annoyances of life became big annoyances. I was finding both my ability to cope and my patience level rapidly declining.

What was happening to me? Why was I feeling this way? I didn't have any answers and I was very concerned. Only later did I realize that all of the above symptoms were classic symptoms of chronic mercury exposure, also known as micromercurialism. And only later did I come to realize that putting in amalgam or drilling out old amalgam exposed the dentist and anyone else in the dental operatory to extremely large amounts of mercury vapor.

About this time a patient came into my office and expressed concern about having a root canal procedure. He said that his naturopathic physician advised him against having a root canal procedure because the bacteria and bacterial toxins present in root canal treated teeth can cause disease elsewhere in the body. He referred to research done in the 1920's linking root canal treated teeth to a host of systemic diseases. Since I had been performing root canal procedures during my entire dental career I set out to research the facts on root canal treated teeth, confident that I would be reporting back to this patient that his fears were unfounded.

My search to prove the safety of the root canal procedure led me to the International Academy of Oral Medicine and Toxicology (IAOMT). This organization has as their stated goal to study the scientific evidence available on the safety of different dental materials and procedures. After a total immersion into both the remote and current research on dental products and procedures, I discovered that my beliefs about many of the currently accepted views on the safety of some dental materials and the safety of some of the dental procedures, such as the root canal procedure, were wrong. The link between dentistry and systemic health was real and absolutely undeniable. Furthermore, much of the most pertinent information I discovered has been known for a long time and seemed to me to have been covered up. I became angry about being misled in my education and I immediately changed the focus of my practice-and totally regained my health.

Claims and Counterclaims

The ADA continues to claim that dental amalgam is safe. The ADA originally claimed that no mercury was released from fillings and that once the mercury was mixed with the silver, copper, tin, and zinc, the mercury was rendered biologically inert. Later, the ADA conceded that some mercury was continuously released from amalgam fillings but supposedly only in toxically insignificant amounts. It claimed that the public is exposed to much higher levels of mercury from fish, air, and water. These statements made by the ADA are simply untrue, and they are a source of ongoing misinformation to the American public, as well as to American dentists. Whether the ADA intends to be misleading is unknown to us. However, since so much of the rest of the world blindly follows the United States in its policies of health care, untold numbers of dentists worldwide also end up following the lead of the ADA. So, what the ADA presents as fact is of great significance in determining how dentistry is practiced over the entire planet. Let's review in greater detail some of the information that continues to be downplayed and apparently even ignored by the ADA.

As mentioned earlier, The United States Environmental Protection Agency (EPA) stated in its 1997 report to Congress that the highest body burden of inorganic mercury comes from amalgam fillings. Let's look at this in more detail. The actual estimated daily dose of mercury exposure from amalgam ranges from 2 to 17 micrograms. This correlates closely to the World Health Organization (WHO) estimate and *Goodman and Gillman's: The Pharmacological Basis of Therapeutics* textbook estimate of 3 to 17 micrograms of mercury exposure per day from amalgam fillings. Currently, the consensus average estimate for absorbed mercury vapor for a person with an average of eight occlusal (chewing surface) fillings is 10 micrograms, which is probably a low estimate. With the United States Public Health Department setting a minimal risk level (MRL) for chronic mercury vapor exposure at 0.28 micrograms /day, the average person with eight chewing surface amalgam fillings and absorbing 10 micrograms of mercury would be over 35 times above the U.S. Public Health MRL for chronic mercury vapor exposure! Why would we continue to place a toxic heavy metal such as mercury into people's mouths when this information is available and there are alternative filling materials?

To answer this question it is of interest to look at the potential economic impact of this situation. As noted earlier in this chapter, the ADA has backed itself into a corner by continuously declaring amalgam completely safe. Even now, in the face of overwhelming evidence to the contrary, this amazing assertion continues to be the ADA's official stance. To admit now that the use of amalgam should be discontinued or even that it *might* be harmful would undoubtedly invite a barrage of lawsuits. Furthermore, if amalgam was banned, the insurance industry would be hit with a major increase in claims, as the alternative fillings are more costly and people would demand that their amalgam fillings be replaced.. It would cost an estimated 250-300 billion dollars to replace all the amalgam fillings currently implanted in the teeth of the American public. It would cost an additional 12-15 billion dollars a year to use alternative non-mercury fillings from this day forward. And since the harmful effects of mercury exposure are characteristically diverse and difficult to diagnose, there would certainly be many people claiming disability because of their fillings. The potential effects of such litigation and disability claims might even be perceived as a threat to the economic stability of the nation. It would be no surprise to find that the parties involved, including the ADA, the insurance companies, and the amalgam manufacturers, would want to perpetuate the myth that mercury amalgam is safe. But decide such issues for yourself. Only the fact that mercury amalgam continually produces toxic mercury vapors is certain. The motivations of the individuals and organizations that continue to support its use are speculative and cannot be known for sure.

Another interesting fact is that mercury amalgam is not officially approved by the Food and Drug Administration (FDA). It is a federal law that any material implanted into the human body for more than 30 days must undergo exhaustive evaluation to determine its safety. The FDA failed to place amalgam in this category by stating that mixed amalgam is the product of the dentist's manufacture in his office and therefore does not need to meet these safety criteria. So this very convoluted reasoning by the FDA means that there are NO safety studies on amalgam!

The fact that mercury amalgam has been used in dentistry for a long time does not mean that it is safe. History is full of products that were once thought to be safe but were eventually proven to be harmful. Asbestos, dioxin, DDT, and Agent Orange are just a few of the products that were once deemed "safe" by the experts. Alcohol and tobacco have also been used for centuries. Such a legacy of long-term use hardly assures that these products are safe and non-toxic which, of course, they are not.

The above discussion on mercury amalgam fillings should serve clear notice that you have to be an educated and motivated consumer of dental services. While this book is primarily directed at the negative impact of dental infections on overall health, the amalgam controversy shows that the stances of official health organizations are not necessarily to be embraced as valid without at least some further examination. Hopefully, in addition to giving you some important information, this book will also serve to make you a more discerning consumer of health care services in general.

4

THE FOCUS IN DENTAL SCHOOL

The Drive to Save Teeth

You are taught in dental school to save teeth. Extraction of a tooth was always the last resort. You are taught that if a tooth was physically and mechanically restorable, regardless of the amount and severity of infection in the tooth and surrounding bone, to try to prevent the tooth from being extracted by performing a root canal procedure. Sometimes the infection could be so severe that a root canal procedure alone would not be sufficient to clear up the immediate signs and symptoms of infection in the surrounding bone. In this case an additional surgical procedure called an apicoectomy was performed. Specifically, an apicoectomy is a procedure where an incision is made in the lower gum tissue to expose the bone covering the apex, or tip, of the tooth root. A hole is then made through the bone to expose the apex of the root and the area of infected bone. As much infected bone as possible is then scraped out, and the tip of the root is usually cut off and sealed. The tip of the root is usually sealed with mercury-containing amalgam. This means that amalgam, a toxic material that outside of the body must be disposed of as hazardous waste, is implanted *directly inside* the body in contact with the jawbone and its blood supply! This procedure results in two clear problems:

1. It leaves a tooth that is still infected since an apicoectomy cannot sterilize the infected area any more effectively than a standard root canal procedure. Bacteria (and sometimes viruses and fungi) can be expected to continue to grow and multiply. These microorganisms and/or their toxic products can then disseminate to other parts of the body over time, just as with a root canal treated tooth.
2. There is a hazardous toxic material, namely mercury-containing dental amalgam, that is often implanted directly inside the bone.

These procedures are all done in the interest of saving a tooth. Why are the possible systemic health consequences of these procedures never taught in dental school? It seems to us that the most compelling reason for this lack of instruction on the health interactions of these procedures is that the ADA gives accreditation to dental schools and therefore dictates curriculum. The ADA has already used its significant resources to largely discredit the brilliant research of Dr. Weston Price that exposed the dangers of the root canal procedure. With Dr. Price's work out of the way, the ADA then proceeded to set treatment standards based on scientific data that was often incomplete, while seeming to ignore additional sources of valid scientific data that did not support its recommendations.

Not only is it unethical to modify scientific fact to support the procedures that you have performed and would like to continue to perform, it is dangerous to patients. This is especially true when a procedure such as a root canal procedure ends up being officially endorsed as a beneficial and worthwhile procedure. The official position of the ADA is that root canals are a safe treatment option for an infected tooth and that any dentist recommending the extraction of an asymptomatic root canal treated tooth should be reported for ethical misconduct! It would seem that the ADA has actually placed serious obstacles in the way of conscientious dentists who place ethical practice and patient welfare at the top of their list of priorities.

Faking It to Graduate

When you are taught to do root canal procedures in dental school the importance of *sterilizing* the root canal is emphasized. This is deemed so important by the dental professors that you are required to take a specimen for culture from the inside of the root canal and send it to the lab to see if any bacteria will grow. Only when the culture comes back negative, meaning that there is no growth of bacteria from the specimen, are you allowed to finish the root canal procedure. When I [RK] trained, many students became frustrated because the culture results kept coming back positive. Because of this, they would often fake this test by placing a sterile collecting swab into the culture media without actually taking a sample from the root canal tooth. This way a negative culture would be guaranteed, and they could then finish the root canal procedure.

But even if the students were conscientious and eventually submitted samples that showed no growth, this was no assurance that the tooth was sterile. For one thing, most of the bacteria infecting root canal treated teeth are anaerobic, meaning that they cannot live or grow in the presence of oxygen. These anaerobic bacteria have to be cultured using specific techniques not ordinarily employed. So, even if the culture came back negative, it would be useless in predicting whether the root canal treated tooth was infected with the more commonly present anaerobic bacteria. Furthermore, it is ridiculous to think that it is possible to sterilize the miles of dentin tubules that can harbor millions of bacteria. It must be emphasized and re-emphasized: *THERE IS NO WAY TO STERILIZE AN INFECTED TOOTH BY PERFORMING A ROOT CANAL PROCEDURE*!

Guarding Your Territory

When the root canal procedure specialists (endodontists) finally accepted that virtually all infected teeth that were given root canal treatments remained infected (a concept that was proven by Dr. Weston Price in the 1920's) they abandoned the practice of attempting to demonstrate a negative culture before completing a root canal procedure. Suddenly, the need to eliminate bacteria and to sterilize the root canal treated tooth in order to assure a successful root canal procedure was abolished.

In defense of this foundational change in treatment goal and philosophy the endodontists stated that although root canal treated teeth may remain infected, the body can "handle" this infection. No longer was sterilization of the tooth, once deemed *vital* to the success of the root canal treatment, given *any* importance in completing the procedure! Further misguiding dentists and patients into believing the root canal procedure to be a safe treatment, the American Association of Endodontists (AAE) state in their Fall/Winter 1994 newsletter that any infection that may spread from a root canal treated tooth will stay around the tooth only and will not travel throughout the rest of the body. This statement has absolutely no medical validity whatsoever and is frankly outrageous given what is known about infections in areas that have good adjacent blood supplies. Just like the ADA, the AAE appears to set its policies to protect the status quo, seemingly without regard for the consequences. Even though the health of many people is at stake, it would nevertheless be amazing to see the AAE question the validity or safety of the a procedure that provides a generous living to most of its members. Organizations rarely attack the primary source of their financial support.

5

IGNORING THE FACTS

The Need for Comprehensive Treatment Plans

When an architect designs a building, all of the structural details must be worked out ahead of time. The construction materials to be used, as well as the functional scenarios to be encountered, must all be taken into consideration to insure that the building will be constructed as safely as possible. As many variables as possible must be studied and analyzed before construction can begin. Although many engineering principles remain constant to all building designs, individual variation must be taken into account for each specific construction project. Factors such as land geology and topography, temperature variations, functional usage, and a host of other factors must be studied in order to design a safe building. The architect must thoroughly understand all of these factors before recommending that the construction begin.

Dentists and physicians must also understand all of the details of the procedures that they perform. It is imperative that they evaluate the complete body of scientific information on a given medical procedure, and take into account individual variability in treatment planning. There is no place for "cookbook" medical or dental care. Dentists are treating intact human beings, not just mouths isolated from their bodies. Patients depend on their dentists to constantly evaluate and re-evaluate the safety of the procedures performed on them in order to tailor their treatment plans to fit them as individuals.

Unfortunately, most dentist's fall very short in elevating the level and quality of care they provide by failing to integrate the broad base of scientific knowledge and the individual health requirements of their patients into their treatment plans. The majority of articles in current dental publications are usually written about new procedural techniques or practice management issues. Almost no attention is given to the general health implications of dental conditions and procedures. Recent rare exceptions are the 1998 reports linking an increased risk of heart disease and stroke to periodontal (gum) disease. These reports probably came to light because medical doctors as well as dentists became aware of these critical mouth-body associations, and one health discipline wanted to report it in the literature ahead of the other health discipline. Furthermore, it certainly can be anticipated that publicizing such information will lead more patients to seek dental treatment to better avoid heart attacks and strokes. The dental community would be expected to want to publicize this discovery since more people seeking treatment for periodontal disease would result in more business and therefore more income for the dentists. This has, in fact, been the case. Not only have the dental journals published numerous articles on this subject, but the general media has published numerous reports on it as well. If, on the other hand, a dental procedure (versus a dental condition such as periodontal disease) were suspected to cause or contribute to disease, it would seem reasonable to expect extensive research into the issue. It would also be appropriate to receive a public warning by the dental organizations about the findings, resulting in a modification, restriction, or elimination of the procedure once the findings had been confirmed. As is the case with dental amalgam placements, this is also not happening with root canal procedures. Most endodontists make all of their income from performing root canals. Root canals are literally *all* they do, day in and day out. Expecting endodontists to individually, or collectively as the AAE, report that root canal procedures are unsafe is simply a colossal and classical conflict of interest, as well as a totally untrue assertion. There should be no complete ignoring or even selective filtration of valid scientific data on the toxicity of root canal treated teeth. You cannot have the fox watching the henhouse and expect the best interests of the hens to be served.

Many general dentists also rely on root canal procedures for a substantial part of their income. Continuing education courses are given on how to do root canal procedures faster and more economically. There are even courses on how to diagnose more teeth in perceived "need" of root canal procedures, further expanding the patient base and the utilization of the procedure. Heroic and expensive treatment procedures are taught in an effort to prevent extraction of infected teeth. Dentists are "conditioned" to save teeth from extraction. Why? Certainly, one reason is that it is a reasonable goal to preserve functional teeth. However, the rest of the body should not have to pay the price. Another reason is that root canal procedures are high-profit dental treatment. In addition, root canal procedures result in dentists performing more crowns and bridges. These procedures also generate large profits in a dental practice, since fewer teeth are extracted and can be the sources of repeated various procedures for years to come.

Nowhere in the current mainstream dental literature were we able to find any publication warning of even possible negative systemic health effects of root canal treated teeth. Yet, every day, potentially damaging health effects are brought about by dental procedures. *Dentistry is hurting people!* So far, the dental profession collectively refuses to accept its sacred responsibility to pursue scientific objectivity, and it refuses to demonstrate the willingness to initiate change when good scientific research so indicates. The AAE does not have the scientific validation on root canal procedures to justify the recommendation that this procedure ever be performed on human beings, or any other animal, for that matter.

Like the architect designing the building, the dentist must be aware of the "landscape"-the general health and other disease processes affecting each individual patient-and have a thorough understanding of all aspects of the procedure before initiating it. This includes all of the implications of the procedure-not just the mechanical aspects but also the clinical consequences. Anybody can be trained to do a root canal. The art and science of dentistry lies in understanding the effects of this procedure on the biochemical, physiological, and immunological systems and how these systems affect the procedure itself. Of course, if these considerations were properly applied to the root canal procedure, it would cease to exist as a dental treatment option.

It is imperative that this multidisciplinary approach be understood and used everyday in clinical dental (and medical) practice settings. Otherwise dentists are merely tooth technicians, dedicated only to performing procedures with an acceptable degree of technical skill but with little, if any, respect and understanding for the complex relationship between these procedures and the overall health and well being of their patients.

Clearly, it is imperative for a dentist to fully understand the possible systemic ramifications of a procedure he or she performs, such as a root canal procedure. It is unconscionable to subject patients to a dental treatment when there are any significant unanswered questions regarding the safety of this treatment. This is especially true when those questions can be easily answered or have already been answered elsewhere. Furthermore, dentists must be willing to honestly and objectively evaluate *all* the available scientific data without regard to economic incentive. A treatment protocol based on selective ignorance is unacceptable.

Seven Important Questions About Root Canal Procedures

Seven questions come to mind that should be answered and understood by all dentists performing root canal procedures. The answers to these questions are important in determining the risk to benefit ratio of a root canal. No dentist should perform a root canal procedure without first knowing the answers to these seven simple but very important questions. Informed consent for a procedure can only be obtained when a patient is given a truthful presentation of all of the available scientific information. This should include an explanation of all known risks, benefits, and alternatives for a root canal. Remember that even though all root canal treated teeth that we have studied are toxic, each patient nevertheless has the right to have such a treatment after receiving a fully informed consent. There do exist rare elderly patients with relatively good health and one or more root canal treated teeth in their mouths. Some people maintain stronger immune systems and are simply able to ward off toxicity much better than others. Even though we would never recommend that any patient be exposed to the chronic toxic insult to their immune system from a root canal treated tooth, the decision still remains with the patient after hearing *all* of the facts (versus the hype).

The Seven Questions on Root Canal Procedures

1. What is the goal of a root canal procedure?

2. Can bacteria remain in ideally treated root canal teeth?
3. Can bacteria or bacterial toxins be released from ideally treated root canal teeth?
4. Can ideally treated root canal teeth cause or contribute to systemic disease?
5. Is there any medical contraindication to a root canal procedure?
6. Is there any clinically restorable tooth on which you would not perform a root canal? If so, what would be the basis for your decision?
7. What is the indication for an apicoectomy and what are you trying to achieve with this procedure? (See Chapter 4)

An inability to answer these questions means that the dentist does not have enough knowledge about how a root canal procedure can be expected to impact on the health of the patient. When the dentist does not know the answers to these questions, the root canal procedure becomes simply a technical process with the patient's health often becoming a casualty.

Some Endodontist "Answers"

These seven questions were presented to two dentists of a prominent Westchester, New York endodontic group. These were the same dentists that attended a lecture by one of this book's authors [RK]. At this event, they attempted to refute most of the scientific data presented with unscientific information. They were also offered a significant collection of clinical data on root canal treated teeth but refused to accept it for review.

After re-contacting these same two dentists, a copy of the above seven questions was FAXed to their office. After about three weeks without a reply, several phone calls were placed to their office. The response of the receptionist was always the same: "The doctor is unavailable and busy with patients but will call you back." The doctor(s) never did respond. No replies to the questions or return phone calls were ever received.

These seven questions were also officially presented to the AAE. An employee of the AAE, who identified herself as the public and professional affairs coordinator of the AAE, had one of the AAE dentists deal with this issue. Over the phone, this dentist was informed that a book on the root canal procedure was being written, and the official position of the AAE on several issues was being sought. He responded that he would be glad to help, and he stated that he had the authority to speak directly for the AAE. He requested that the questions be FAXed to him and that he would reply in about a week. When no follow-up phone call from this dentist was received, he was recontacted. He now asked what the intentions of the book were. He was advised that the book was aimed at informing the public about the truth regarding root canal procedures. He said that the board of directors at the AAE had some legal issues to work out before the questions could be answered. Again a follow-up call was promised for the following week. And again, no call was received. After attempting one more time to contact him, a message was left, and a return call was finally received from a lady who identified herself as an assistant director of the AAE. She said that the AAE was refusing to comment on the seven questions that were presented! She even commented that "the AAE is not here to help you write a book." After she said that the AAE would freely supply such information to the general public, she was told that this *was* an inquiry from a member of the public and that answers were being sought regarding the AAE's declared area of expertise. She continued to decline comment and the conversation ended abruptly. What are these dentists and the American Academy of Endodontics afraid of?

Every patient scheduled for a root canal procedure should be advised to ask their dentist these seven questions. Also, seek the answers directly from the AAE, and see for yourself how little valid scientific information and how few (if any) published scientific articles you receive. In fact, the AAE has *no* scientific article to refute the work of Weston Price and E.C. Rosenow, although they claim that they do. None of the articles offered by the AAE effectively disproves the focal infection concept or the negative health effects of root canal treated teeth.

You have a right to know the answers. It just might be tough to know which answers are correct. Demand to see the scientific evidence for all of the answers you are given. If such evidence is not forthcoming, be suspicious and more demanding, not less.

6

THE DIRECT EVIDENCE

Sterile Instruments, Infected Teeth

Today, most dental offices practice meticulous sterilization techniques in the attempt to have good infection control. In fact, all dental office employees in the state of New York are required to attend an infection control course every four years. Patients expect to see protective coverings on objects such as the dental light handles changed between patients. Instruments are thoroughly scrubbed and sterilized after each use, and kept wrapped in sterile packets. The dentist and dental assistant both wear gloves and masks to help prevent any transmission of infectious agents. The emphasis on sterile technique is well accepted by both the general public and dentists alike.

It is important for all dental offices to ensure that the water that runs through the dental equipment is free of microorganisms. The small tubing that leads to the dental drills, the air/water sprayer that dentists use to wash and dry teeth, and the unit that fills the cup for rinsing can all collect large amounts of bacteria and other microbes. In fact, an investigative report on a television news magazine showed that water from a toilet was cleaner and contained less bacteria that the water coming out of much of the dental equipment tested!

The explanation for this problem is the small diameter of the tubing supplying water to the dental equipment as well as the "suck back" of water that occurs from the patient back into the dental equipment such as the dental drill. Saliva from patient to patient can be sucked back into the tubing leading to cross-contamination. Also, the small volume of water flowing through the dental lines does not allow flushing out of the bacteria. And to further complicate matters, the bacteria produce a bio-film, which is a sticky accumulation of bacteria within the water lines. Be sure your dentist has added filtration units and anti-"suck back" devices to the dental equipment.

With all of the proper sterilization procedures in place, the risk of transmitting any disease from dentist or dental assistant to a patient is close to zero. Furthermore, dentistry has done a tremendous job eliminating cross-contamination of microorganisms between patients. In fact, most dental procedures are designed to eliminate bacteria that cause disease. When a filling procedure is performed, the decayed part of the tooth along with the decay-causing bacteria is removed and a filling is then placed to prevent re-infection and further decay. Failure to remove all of the decay, and therefore all of the decay-causing bacteria, will result in the continuation of the decay process. Similarly, a major component of periodontal (gum) treatment is the elimination of the pathogenic microorganisms that cause this condition. If the microorganisms are not eliminated, then the periodontal disease continues. So, it is important to prevent the spread of disease from one patient to another by proper sterilization techniques, just as it is important to eliminate the disease-causing bacteria in the dental procedures.

But what if one of the dental procedures fails to meet these criteria of pathogenic bacterial elimination? Can such a procedure be deemed successful? Is this procedure in the best interest of the patient's overall health? Is this procedure at all consistent with the critical concept of proper sterile technique?

Such a procedure is the root canal procedure. Following every such procedure on an infected tooth, the same bacteria that caused the infection in the first place remain in the porous dentin tubules. As was described earlier, there is currently no way to sterilize infected teeth while they are still in the jawbone; they all remain infected after the root canal procedures. So, despite all of dentistry's efforts to utilize sterile instruments, in performing a root canal procedure the original infection within the treated tooth will remain. The original goal of the procedure, namely the elimination of bacteria from an infected tooth, cannot be met and has never been met. Even if all of the instruments used are sterile, a tooth infected before a root canal procedure will still be infected after a root canal procedure. While the meticulous dentist might not necessarily be introducing any new infectious agents at the time of the procedure, many such organisms are still left behind.

Seeing and Smelling Is Believing

Extractions of root canal treated teeth are always enlightening events for the patients having the extractions. If the patients are not totally convinced of the need for extraction before the procedure, they most certainly are convinced after the procedure. I [RK] make it a point to show the patient the tooth after the extraction. Many times it is discolored, with infected tissue around the tip of the root. I also show them the mushy or discolored diseased bone that is removed from the extraction socket. But the most convincing moment comes when I let the curious patient smell the extracted tooth. It stinks! The odor of dead, necrotic, and infected tissue is an unforgettable smell. My dental assistant once described an extracted root canal treated tooth as smelling like a dead mouse that had been decomposing for a while. (By contrast, healthy teeth extracted for reasons such as braces have normal color and no foul odor. They are not infected, and therefore have no associated dead and rotting tissue.) I then ask the patient if they would like to have that infected, smelly tooth put back into their body and the answer is always an emphatic "NO WAY!" Yet, similar root canal treated teeth remain in the mouths of people for many years, and many more new root canal procedures are performed every day. Dr. John Hunter was a prominent physician who many years ago described a root canal treated tooth restored with a gold crown in this way: "A devitalized tooth (root canal treated tooth) is like a sea of sepsis (infection) under a mausoleum of gold." It is doubtful that Dr. Hunter would be at all amazed by the sights and smells of extracted root canal treated teeth.

Prevention Versus Prescription

If virtually all root canal treated teeth are infected with microorganisms then why isn't everyone with a root canal treated tooth sick? To answer this question we must first explore our current perspectives on health and disease.

Medicine today seeks to cure disease with a "cookbook" approach to diagnosis and treatment. First, a patient presents to the physician with a list of symptoms. Then the doctor performs a physical examination and takes note of clinical signs and symptoms. Laboratory tests and x-ray studies may be ordered. Finally, a diagnosis is made based upon the patient's described symptoms and the doctor's physical exam and workup. The diagnosed "disease" is given a name and is then treated, usually with drugs or surgery.

Most medicine today is practiced this way. Our health care system is really a "disease care" system. Doctors are not trained to maintain health but rather are trained to treat disease, and sometimes just the *symptoms* of disease. The evolution of health care to the sub-specialty level, with doctors that specialize in treating body parts (for example, a cardiologist for the heart or a pulmonologist for the lung), along with treatment protocols largely dictated by insurance companies, has forced physicians to practice a reactionary form of medicine. If a given patient has disease A, then the appropriate drug to treat disease A is prescribed. It seems that anticipation and prevention of disease are rarely considered and even more rarely emphasized in the medical training programs. Medicine has largely been reduced to a state of reaction to what is already there and presenting itself as symptoms.

Life is a Many-Splendored Thing

The problem is that we do not always look for the factors that make the person susceptible to disease in the first place. What factors weaken the body, making it initially vulnerable to illness?

Our state of health is not linear. Physics can easily define linear equations such as distance equals velocity multiplied by time. Many things can be explained in linear terms, meaning that a direct correlation can be made between the degree to which a factor is present and the degree of effect that factor has on a measurable system. The problem is that most things do not fit linear equations. The chaos theory dominates our physical surroundings. The chaos theory states that most events have too many variables to be explained in linear terms. Weather, for example, follows the principles of the chaos theory. There are too many variables in creating weather patterns to accurately predict weather conditions far in advance. There are simply no linear equations to take into account all of the variables that create weather.

A drop of water hangs from the lip of a faucet and finally drips off. This seems like a simple event. But try to devise a mathematical formula to predict how the drop of water will leave the faucet and suddenly the formula becomes extremely complex. Just like weather, there are too many variables to describe this action in linear terms.

The human body, in either disease or health, is also too complex to treat in linear terms. Although medicine has been successful in treating some diseases by closely observing cause-and-effect, many other disease states fail to conform to this way of thinking. In order to fully understand the intricacies of health and disease states we must look at all the aspects of a person's life.

The body is a marvelously complex biochemical organism. Like a symphony orchestra, when all of the instruments are perfectly tuned and the musicians are playing flawlessly, the concert hall is filled with beautiful music. Similarly, when all of the biochemical processes in the body are functioning at peak performance, we are free from disease and maintain a state of optimum health. We feel great when our bodies are performing like a flawlessly executed concerto.

But what if several of the instruments in the orchestra suddenly start playing slightly out of tune? The concert would surely continue with maybe only a handful of the audience noticing the degradation of the music. Now let's imagine that a few more instruments start playing erratically. The conductor may notice the problem and try to correct it. Nevertheless, even with a decline in the quality of the performance the concert continues. It won't be until one instrument begins to play so erratically as to stand out from the rest of the orchestra, or until all of the instruments play somewhat erratically, that the music ceases to reasonably resemble an identifiable symphony..

The changes may be subtle at first. But if left to continue and multiply, the end result is a complete breakdown of the musical performance.

The human body is much like a symphony orchestra, only incredibly more complex. With biochemical processes all working at peak efficiency we function in a state of health. However, when some of the biological processes start to falter due to disease and toxicity, we are no longer performing at our optimum level. We may not notice the subtle changes at first but these changes can eventually have an effect on our overall state of health. Our bodies have a tremendous ability to heal themselves if given a chance, and our adaptive abilities are superb. Nevertheless, if we continue to damage the biochemical processes that are crucial to life, we may find that the body can no longer repair itself and we become susceptible to disease.

Variable Immune System Strength

There may be one major event that triggers disease, or there may be many small events that wear down one or more of the many systems in the body, most significantly the immune system.

A boxer in a fight can be knocked down in the first round with a knockout punch. Or, a boxer can go 15 rounds with constant jabs to the head. Finally, in the 15th round he takes a jab and is knocked out cold. Was it the last jab that knocked him out or was it the culmination of 15 rounds of jabs that wore him down?

The same considerations hold true for the human body. Our health care providers must look deeper for the cause of a disease instead of just treating its symptoms. They must learn to cultivate a state of health rather than just treat a state of disease. They must understand what constitutes optimal health and then help patients to reach this goal. The body cannot be treated as a pile of parts. Although there may *rarely* be just one cause for a disease state, more than likely there are numerous factors, all working in concert, contributing to clinical illness. Everything in our body is linked. Rather than to address isolated aspects of the body, it is ultimately far more effective to address the body as a complete entity.

So how does this relate to a root canal procedure? Root canal treated teeth are always infected, usually immediately following the procedure but always eventually. The bacteria present in root canal treated teeth can vary from mildly pathogenic to highly pathogenic. These bacteria and/or their toxins may be released from the root canal treated teeth in large or small quantities. The ability of the body's immune system to cope with this assault may be adequate to prevent disease or it may not. If the immune system can handle this infection for the moment, there may not be any outward signs of disease. However, if the immune system is unable to fully counteract the bacteria or bacterial toxins, then subtle changes in a person's health can be expected to develop. This toxic stress also leads to a weakened immune state making the body susceptible to other disease processes and further breakdown. Eventually, a person will end up developing a significant disease such as cancer, heart disease, or some other degenerative disease. Surely, there may be other more recent factors that may have been the "straw that broke the camel's back." Or maybe, when the immune system has already been severely weakened, the toxicity from the root canal treated tooth can be strong enough to be a potential knockout punch to the immune system and to bring about a rapid appearance of toxin-induced disease.

All of this means that different people respond differently to the same immunologic stress. Some people will get sick very rapidly after a root canal procedure, and other people will fight both the acute and chronic stress of the root canal more effectively for much longer periods of time. This means that the appearance of a disease secondary to the immune stress from a root canal treated tooth may occur months or even *many years* later! This is a primary reason why so many root canal treated teeth are not suspected of being the disease-causing culprits. If the root canal procedure was performed years or even decades earlier, neither the typical physician nor the typical dentist can conceive that it could possibly relate to the current illness. The trouble is, when the overtaxed immune system finally stops coping, the disease will then appear. And many people can cope with chronic immune stress for years.

Conditions Favoring Toxicity

Root canal treated teeth can contain a wide variety of microorganisms including bacteria, viruses and fungi. It is important to always consider the many potential interactions that such microorganisms can have with the different cells in the body. There are many beneficial interactions that the human body can have with microbes, yet there are probably even more pathogenic, or disease-producing, interactions that microbes can have in the body.

Some microbes that are normally beneficial, or at least nonpathogenic may *become* pathogenic depending upon their immediate surroundings inside the body. Many dentists claim that the body is "full" of bacteria and that the body can "handle" any bacteria normally left behind in a root canal treated tooth. Just because one part of the body (such as the inside of the mouth) may be normally teeming with bacteria in a healthy body does not mean that all of the other parts of the body (such as the inner pulp of a tooth) can tolerate such a bacterial presence. The pulp of any tooth *MUST* be sterile. *Not even the limited presence of pathogenic bacteria or other microbes is acceptable.*

Remember that until it was re-established that root canal treated teeth remained infected (confirming the work of Price and Rosenow), a root canal procedure was only considered effective if *all* bacteria were eliminated. Now that we know that you simply cannot eliminate all bacteria from the root canal treated pulp, the dental establishment has changed their definition of a "successful" root canal procedure. With or without inflammation, any bacteria remaining in a root canal treated pulp represents an unacceptable presence. Furthermore, this infection will remain chronic and toxic as long as the root canal treated tooth remains in the mouth and does not get properly extracted. The presence of bacteria in the root canal treated tooth, unlike in the environment of the mouth itself, represents a pathological condition that persists for as long as the root canal treated tooth stays in the jawbone.

There is no symbiosis or benefit that will ever result from the presence of bacteria in an environment that is designed to remain absolutely sterile. To the contrary, such a bacterial symbiotic relationship can be found inside our intestines. These "friendly" bacteria inside our gut participate in a number of interactions in the proper digestion of our food and the promotion of normal physiology and good health. These bacteria are helpful to our body and do not cause disease. However, when the immediate environment of these symbiotic bacteria is disrupted and altered, the proliferation of pathogenic bacteria can rapidly ensue, and the potential for the development of disease results. Interestingly, the pathogenic bacteria may be new invaders, or they may result from "friendly" bacteria subjected to a hostile environment (such as the toxic transformation of mouth bacteria when trapped inside a root canal treated pulp without oxygen). But remember that, unlike in the intestine, there can never be any normal growth of "friendly" bacteria inside a tooth pulp.

All life, regardless of its complexity, looks for ways to survive and reproduce. The bacteria infecting root canal treated teeth are no different. They will do anything in their power to proliferate. Although most of them prefer an environment containing oxygen, they will mutate and survive in oxygen-depleted conditions rather than just die. In so adapting, they typically become pathogenic in the process. How pathogenic they become depends on the type of bacteria. Root canal treated teeth have had well over 100 different types of bacteria isolated from them, and the types of toxins produced and the disease states induced can vary substantially with the bacteria type.

This is completely consistent with the results of Dr. Price's research discussed in Chapter 2.

Bacteria from root canal treated teeth that have found their way from the pulp to the surrounding bone have clever defense mechanisms to avoid attack by the immune system. For one thing, these bacteria release chemicals that effectively block the process called chemotaxis, which allows the disease-fighting white blood cells to be attracted to the infected site. Not all the "reinforcements" in the world can beat an invader if they cannot reach the invader in the first place. Another defense mechanism involves the bacteria building a "fortress" in the bone in which they can effectively "hide" from the immune system. One way in which they do this is by invading the small blood vessels called capillaries and multiplying along the inside of the blood vessel in what is called a biofilm. In this biofilm the bacteria adhere to the walls of these capillaries by secreting a sticky material called glycocalix. The bacterial colonies grow from the capillary wall out until they effectively block off the entire capillary. Once this blockage occurs, no blood can travel through the capillary. Bone cells that receive their blood supply from such blocked capillaries then become cut off from adequate blood supply and can die. However, the bacteria living in this bone will adapt to the decreased blood supply and subsequently decreased oxygen and nutrient supply, establishing their own little niche. They also effectively shield themselves even further from the immune system, since the blood supply to the site of infection has become even more severely diminished.

A good blood supply is absolutely essential for proper immune access to any infected tissue. It is interesting to note that some root canal treated teeth cause a large amount of swelling, pus, and inflammation in the surrounding tissue indicating that the body is mounting a more pronounced attack on the infection than is usually seen. Dr. Price found that this type of patient, one who mounts a strong immune response, showed less systemic disease from the presence of the root canal treated teeth than the patient who showed little evidence of local infection. The patient who mounted little or no immune response and showed non-existent or only slight pathological signs and symptoms around their root canal treated teeth often had *more* severe systemic complications and disease. Basically, the root canal treated teeth that looked the best and felt the best were actually the most toxic! This makes sense since the bacteria are free to "set up shop," survive, and disseminate more bacteria and bacterial toxins throughout the body when the immune system is not mounting its classic inflammatory response to infection. An active immune response indicates that the body is clearly "seeing" and fighting the infection. Although the local clinical manifestations of an active immune response may at first appear to indicate a more severe systemic problem, many times it is the asymptomatic root canal treated tooth that may be doing the most damage to the body. This makes it very difficult to diagnose which root canal treated tooth may be causing the most clinical harm. We absolutely *cannot* rely on local signs and symptoms of the tooth in question to always indicate the potential for systemic effects.

Additional Concepts of Infection

Every organism has an intelligence, and the bacterium is no exception. The complexity of the pathogenic relationship between some bacteria and our bodies is only beginning to be understood. We have made substantial progress in understanding the purely biological/chemical interactions of infection although much of this appears to remain unacknowledged by many in dentistry and medicine. We must now explore the possible disruptions that infected teeth can cause to the normal energy flow in the body.

Many of us are aware of acupuncture and the concept of energy flowing through pathways called meridians. The body has an energy flow, and in eastern philosophy this is called qi. Many eastern philosophies believe that in order to maintain health it is imperative to maintain the flow of qi, as qi is viewed as the life force itself. If we disrupt this flow of qi, the body reacts much like a forest when a river to it gets partially dammed up-the forest becomes chronically malnourished. In a similar fashion, when the normal and healthy energy flow in the body is compromised, this will ultimately cause disease or malfunction. A root canal treated tooth is a functionally dead, yet chronically diseased body part. Because it is no longer alive it is not positively contributing to the enhancement of qi in the body. In fact, this dead and infected tooth may well block the natural flow of qi. And as the bacteria and their toxins make their way from a root canal treated tooth throughout the body, the compromise of normal energy flow is probably yet another negative effect, in addition to the more traditionally recognized results of toxicity.

There are also theories that each tooth is connected to a specific body part or area by its energy meridian. An infection in a tooth may cause a disease process to occur in its corresponding target tissue along its meridian. While this tooth correlation is not absolute, a high degree of clinically practical correlation with these meridian links does appear to exist. At the very least, there are some remote clinical correlations of body tissue response to tooth extractions that are not readily explained in traditional physiological and pathological terms.

The Fatally Flawed Root Canal Procedure: An Unreachable Primary Goal

According to the endodontists, the goal of a root canal procedure is the elimination of infection in the tooth along with the sealing of the root canal system to prevent leakage and, supposedly, subsequent re-infection. Currently, by its own admission, the American Academy of Endodontists acknowledges that most root canal treated teeth remain infected. Logically, then, the Academy is stating that the very goal of a root canal procedure, the eradication of infection, is rarely met. Furthermore, the current materials used to fill the evacuated root canal spaces do not make a perfect seal and thus can always be expected to leak. This leakage allows bacteria and their toxins access to the bloodstream with subsequent dissemination to the rest of the body. The filling materials used to seal an evacuated root canal space have a wax content that *always* shrinks away from the walls of the canal after placement, setting, and cooling. This consistently sets the stage for re-infection and leakage, assuming the bacteria was ever eliminated in the first place. However, as noted earlier, this is not likely ever to occur with the routine sterilization procedures used in the root canal procedure.

In addition, I [RK] have found that nearly all root canal treated teeth that I have extracted are not completely cleaned of the dead and infected pulp tissue, and have confirmed this by histological pathology. This should come as no surprise. The root canal procedure in which the pulp tissue is reamed out is an imprecise and blind procedure at best. There is no conceivable way that this crude evacuation of pulp tissue, which can never be done under direct visualization, represents a precise and complete removal of all the infected tissue. Furthermore, a significant portion of the area targeted for evacuation is physically far beyond the reach of the dental routing tools. And even if the pulp tissue was somehow 100% removed, the routing tools cannot scrape out the miles (literally!) of the surrounding infected dentin tubules that always harbor bacteria when the pulp is infected. *Therefore, the standard root canal procedure can never completely eliminate the presence of bacteria in the dentin tubules, and the standard sealing materials can never completely prevent the migration and leakage of bacteria and their metabolic toxins to the remainder of the tooth and then to the rest of the body.*

Pathology reports from extracted root canal treated teeth also typically reflect the presence of infected and dead tissue that had never been completely removed from the main, central canal inside the tooth. Therefore, if we know that even the *most accessible* internal part of the tooth cannot be completely cleaned in most cases, it is obvious that the main bulk of the tooth surrounding this canal that is *not accessible* during a root canal procedure must always remain infected. This part of the tooth is comprised of the laterally radiating accessory canals and the innumerable, microscopic dentin tubules. This further establishes that the goal of a root canal procedure, the elimination of bacteria and infection, can never be reached when the tooth is infected at the outset, which is very often the primary indication for performing the root canal procedure in the first place.

So how is it really determined whether a root canal procedure is a success or a failure? Clearly, the methods used must be indirect since the actual elimination of bacteria in the tooth is never really achieved, and most endodontists can only hope to imply that the bacteria have been eradicated. Although often used to support a claim of a sterile pulp or central tooth canal, an x-ray evaluation can only detect the most obvious of abscesses in a tooth. An x-ray can never detect the chronic harboring of bacteria in the dentin tubules along with the metabolic toxins that they chronically produce. Toxins and bacteria will never make a shadow on an x-ray. Furthermore, although pain can be an indicator of infection, the lack of pain is no assurance that a chronic, low-grade infection with the production of toxins is not present. As we described earlier, pain is not always present, even in the most toxic of root canal treated teeth. In fact, as noted earlier, the root canal treated teeth that have the least discomfort and associated symptoms are typically the most toxic. Just as in the example of women with infected tampons and toxic shock syndrome, severely toxic and even fatal consequences can occur in the absence of pain at the site of toxin production. In toxic shock syndrome this site is the infected tampon, and in the dental patient this site is the toxic root canal treated tooth that only appears to be free of infection.

Testing for Toxins

A simple screening test to help determine the extent of toxicity in some root canal treated teeth and other dental conditions has been developed by Dr. Boyd Haley and Dr. Curt Pendergrass of the University of Kentucky. This test is quick, painless, and non-invasive, and it can be done in the dental office. The test involves the collection of small amounts of fluid, called gingival crevicular fluid (GCF) from the space between the tooth and the surrounding gum tissue, or gingiva. Bacterial toxins associated with this tooth will often be found in this fluid. This fluid is evaluated by testing how much these toxins inhibit the function of six selected, key enzymes that are directly involved in the production and metabolism of energy by the body. A highly toxic tooth will release potent toxins that will neutralize one or more of these important enzymes in the body. If these toxins significantly disrupt the function of these energy-related enzymes, then it is considered likely that they are also disrupting other critical enzymes in the body. This would also imply that the dental toxins were likely exerting additional non-enzymatic toxic effects on a wide variety of the tissues in the body.

Thus, it is possible to obtain some measure of toxicity from a given tooth. However, it is very critical to emphasize that it is *not* clear whether all toxic teeth will produce GCF samples that will prove to be toxic by this test. Still only an investigational tool, this screening test will produce both false negative and false positive tests. Periodontal disease can give a false positive result for a deep tooth infection when only the gums are infected, since the bacterial toxins associated with infected gums can also inhibit the enzymes in the test. In addition, a false negative result may occur if the toxins remain deep in the infected bone and do not communicate with the GCF for detection. This test promises to provide an increased understanding of the toxicology of the mouth and its infective conditions. However, a negative GCF test for the presence of toxins should *NEVER* be used to conclude that a given root canal treated tooth is toxin-free. To date, *all* root canal treated teeth that have been extracted and submitted for toxicology studies have proven to be very toxic. Current research is being conducted to try to further define the possibilities as well as the limitations of this promising technology.

Desperately Seeking Sterility

Many dentists who are aware of the toxicity of the root canal procedure have been searching for methods to both render root canal treated teeth sterile and then establish a leak-proof seal in the main canal. Most commonly, these dentists try to achieve these goals with a dental laser and a filling material known by the trade name, Biocalex. The laser is intended to kill the bacteria present in the infected tooth, and the Biocalex sealer is intended to both kill bacteria and extend a limited distance into the dentin tubules with a resultant leak-proof seal. These are admirable goals, and it would be fantastic if these goals could be achieved. Unfortunately these goals are never realized with these agents, and the root canal procedure remains an inherently toxic, fatally flawed procedure, regardless of the materials and methods utilized.

But why wouldn't a laser and a filling material like Biocalex achieve these goals? We all think of lasers as a treatment modality with unlimited potential. Certainly, lasers have already done many fantastic things and undoubtedly will continue to have even more impressive applications over time in all areas of science, including medicine and dentistry. However, a laser works according to scientific, not mystical, principles, and there are straightforward, logical reasons why it cannot sterilize a root canal treated tooth.

The root of a tooth has a main canal that travels the length of the tooth. Many times this canal is also curved, and occasionally it branches, subdividing into separate canals. The fiber of the laser delivery system only delivers the laser light from its tip. Laser light travels in a straight line, with very little dissipation or scatter over distance, as occurs when a more traditional light source, such as a flashlight, is used. If you ever attended a concert and observed the laser lights, you can see that they are perfectly straight. A laser pointer at a lecture also demonstrates how focused, straight, and unscattered laser light is. In fact, you cannot get a straighter line than that produced by a laser. This inherent straightness of laser light is directly incompatible with the inherently curved and multifaceted internal configuration of a tooth pulp. It is absolutely impossible to insert a laser into the main canal of a root canal treated tooth and expect the laser light to extend laterally into the body of the tooth and kill the bacteria in the dentin tubules. Similarly, a laser is absolutely incapable of following any curve at all that is present in the primary canal or in any of the lateral accessory canals. Just as significantly, you cannot kill the bacteria in the periodontal ligament surrounding the tooth or those bacteria that are often found in the bone at the apex of the tooth, as this area simply cannot be accessed by light from any source.

Dentists will actually proclaim that because they see the red aiming laser light shining "through" the tooth, they are reassured that the laser is disinfecting the entire tooth. What they are in fact seeing is the red glow emanating from around the tubular laser conduit and its tip, as well as the reflected and refracted light that would make the entire tooth "glow" regardless of the primary light source. This could be considered "laser-associated" light, but it is not remotely the same light as that contained in the laser beam itself. Shine an ordinary laser pointer inside a small crystal, and the whole structure will glow, but only the part of the crystal directly in front of the laser beam will receive the full effect of the concentrated beam. Similarly, a laser pointer pressed against your cheek will also make part of the surrounding cheek not directly in the path of the laser beam glow a bit. And so it is with the tooth as well. It is the very nature of light to continue to bounce off of reflective surfaces and be bent and transmitted through refractive surfaces. But once any reflection or refraction has occurred, the concentrated effects of the original laser light have been lost. It is impossible to direct laser light toward all aspects of the internal tooth as well as to reach the surrounding infected bone in order to accomplish sterilization.

A simple experiment further illustrates this concept. An extracted tooth can be prepared for a root canal procedure just as though it were still in the mouth. One such tooth was given a complete root canal procedure with the cleaning and shaping of the canal performed exactly as would be done in the mouth. Dental plaque samples, which contain live bacteria, were then placed on the outside root surface for the full length of this treated tooth. The tooth was then treated with a dental laser that was set on 15 watts, which is about *ten* times the energy that would be used on an actual tooth inside the mouth. Furthermore, this laser treatment was extended for roughly *ten* times the recommended exposure time. This translates to a laser treatment roughly 100-fold more intense than is typically administered in the mouth. The plaque samples were then retrieved for examination under a microscope. If the laser sterilized the tooth to the outside perimeter, then no live bacteria should be visible. Instead, microscopic examination revealed a host of bacteria that were very much alive. It appeared that the laser had no detectable effect on these plaque-associated bacteria. The laser undoubtedly did what it could be expected to do and nothing more: sterilize only that part of the tooth that was directly in front of the laser beam. Areas "lit up" by reflected laser light showed no sterilization effect, as scientific logic would predict. It should be obvious now how the presence of some curvature in the main canal can prevent even the complete sterilization of that part of the tooth, which is far more accessible than the lateral canals and the dentin tubules.

One other important point needs to be made concerning the ongoing quest to find a way to "sterilize" a root canal treated tooth. Even if a technology could be found that could truly eradicate all of the bacteria in a root canal treated tooth's pulp area, dentin tubules, periodontal ligament, and surrounding infected bone and socket structures, the resulting sterile state would only be very short-lived. As touched upon earlier in this book, the very nature of the root canal procedure, which destroys the internal contents and blood supply of the tooth, effectively blocks immune system function in the core of that tooth by blocking immune system access. When immune access is impeded in this fashion, bacteria are free to be reintroduced into the tooth and to re-colonize the tooth in fairly short order. The mouth has an incredible abundance of microorganisms in it, and without an intact immune system with good access to all parts of the largely dead and non-viable root canal treated tooth, core infection becomes quickly re-established. Re-infection, of course, requires the almost inconceivable result that the root canal treated tooth could even be rendered sterile in the first place.

The only conceivable *theoretical* fashion in which a root canal treated tooth could be "saved" would be to have a method of tooth and tooth socket sterilization that could be easily and non-invasively reapplied on a regular basis. None of the current attempts to sterilize a root canal treated tooth are even effective on a *one-time* basis using a very *invasive* approach. Never say never, perhaps, but the prospects for making the root canal treated tooth a permanently non-toxic entity inside the mouth remain extremely remote.

Now let's look at sealing agents used after a root canal procedure. Gutta-percha, the commonly used waxy substance, is known to shrink away from the opposing tooth canal surfaces after it has been placed. But what about Biocalex as a root canal sealer? Biocalex is a calcium oxide paste that converts to calcium carbonate in the evacuated root canal space. Proponents of Biocalex claim that it seeks out moisture in the tooth and expands somewhat into the lateral canals and dentin tubules, thereby preventing leakage. Furthermore, the pH of Biocalex is very high meaning that it is very alkaline. This alkaline pH can also inhibit the growth of bacteria. These properties of Biocalex would appear to be very desirable, and Biocalex would appear to be a better root canal filling material than gutta-percha. However, the ability of Biocalex to completely seal off the main canal and inhibit bacterial growth still does not reconcile with the clinical and laboratory findings of individuals with Biocalex-filled root canal treated teeth. Like gutta percha-filled root canal spaces, Biocalex-filled teeth have also proved to be highly toxic on the Haley-Pendergrass toxicity test for enzyme inhibition upon extraction.

Just as would be expected in a "regular" root canal treated tooth filled with gutta percha, these extracted teeth that had been filled with Biocalex also demonstrate osteomyelitis of the surrounding bone on pathology reports. Osteomyelitis is inflamed bone that is nearly always infected. This would indicate that Biocalex does not make the tooth non-toxic, and it does not solve the problem of preventing the infection of supporting bone.

Unfortunately, the availability of Biocalex seems to give many dentists who are reluctant or unwilling to stop doing root canal procedures an excuse to continue doing them. Remember how toxic the toxins from root canal treated teeth are. More toxic than even botulism against many of the enzymes tested, it takes only very tiny amounts of these toxins to cause and sustain many different disease processes. Reducing the amount of toxicity produced or having a lesser degree of toxicity leaking out of the inner tooth, to even the smallest degree, may seem like positive goals. But consider a hypothetical situation: If an atomic bomb with one-tenth the power of a typical atomic bomb to fell on you, the ultimate devastation would still be the same. Having a mouth filled with root canal treated teeth that have one-tenth the toxicity than that seen with typical root canal treated teeth will be just as harmful to you clinically as the "fully" toxic root canals. And that assumes that a root canal treated tooth filled with Biocalex is really "less" toxic than a typical root canal treated tooth, which is far from clearly being the case.

The real damage of Biocalex as a root canal filling material comes from this idea of "lessened" toxicity. This has resulted in many dentists continuing to perform a procedure that is intrinsically and fatally flawed, with nearly universal effects on general health. You won't survive one tenth of an atomic bomb blast, and your immune system will be severely traumatized by one tenth of the toxicity of a typical root canal treated tooth. These toxins are simply so potent that no rationalization (such as saving the tooth at all cost), should allow the performance of a root canal procedure, no matter what the filling material. It also is very important to emphasize that Biocalex doesn't prevent or resolve the infection of the periodontal ligament and surrounding bone.

There is also another important concern that is unique to the root canal treated tooth filled with Biocalex. Root canal treated teeth filled with gutta percha classically have a very characteristic, easy-to-identify appearance on x-ray. There are an increasing number of people today who seek to have their root canal treated teeth extracted in order to lessen their toxin exposure and hopefully improve their medical conditions. Many alternative-oriented physicians feel that cancer and other advanced degenerative diseases simply will not respond positively as long as something as toxic as a root canal treated tooth remains in the body. Dr. Josef Issels found that fully 98%

of his adult cancer patients had between two and ten "dead" teeth. And although other circumstances could account for a "dead" tooth, Dr. Issels considered all root canal treated teeth to be "dead"; he required their extraction before proceeding with any of his cancer therapies. Biocalex has the added disadvantage of being very difficult, if not impossible, to routinely identify on an x-ray unless the tooth has had another substance added to it to make it more visible on x-ray. Root canal spaces filled with gutta percha, however, show up very prominently on x-ray. Many sick people in the future who have Biocalex-filled root canals and want all possible infected teeth extracted will often end up with such root canal treated teeth going completely undetected. Dental records are often lost or not easily located; x-rays in conjunction with a clinical examination often are the only way to determine which teeth are infected and continuing to harm a patient's immune system thus preventing clinical improvement or recovery. Hopefully a substance will eventually be developed to negate the toxicity of a root canal treated tooth; Biocalex is definitely not that substance.

Recently, at a meeting of alternatively-oriented dentists, a prominent dentist who is a well-known anti-mercury amalgam spokesperson but who very much favors the use of Biocalex as a root canal filling material gave a presentation on whether root canal procedures should continue to be performed. Although he did not mention Biocalex by name, he presented information on generic calcium oxide, and made comparisons to conventional root canal filling material. He then went on to editorialize about dentists who believe that no root canal procedures should ever be performed. He said that dentists that advise extraction of all infected teeth and do not believe that any endodontic procedure is biocompatible will surely be targeted by their dental boards for investigation. He went on to say that dentists should seriously consider the practical consequences of not performing a root canal while instead recommending extraction of all infected teeth. He warned that the revocation of a dental license will render a dentist incapable of helping other patients and will cause a loss of income to the dentist's family. The irony here is that the same negative consequences have occurred and continue to occur to dentists that do not place mercury amalgam fillings. One wonders if this dentist would support the use of amalgam for the same reasons that he advised against the total elimination of root canal procedures. Furthermore, this dentist appears to have a very basic conflict of interest in his promotion of a procedure from which he may directly benefit financially-his company imported and distributed Biocalex. To make it worse, his position as a lecturer to the largest organized group of alternatively oriented dentists gives him far too much credibility in supporting the ongoing performance of this flawed and toxic procedure.

There is no question, then, that there does not yet exist a way to make root canal treated teeth sterile and non-toxic. Furthermore, the nature of the root canal procedure itself makes it inconceivable that it could ever be performed in a sterile and non-toxic fashion. Certainly dental laser treatment and Biocalex may well represent minor improvements over the usual use of gutta-percha as a root canal space filling. However, do not think that just because a technique is new and sounds "high-tech", it must necessarily be effective. The studies to date have proven that this is not the case.

7

HIDDEN GANGRENE: THE CAVITATION

Overview

While the title of this chapter may seem a bit alarming and even a bit incredible, it is no exaggeration. A cavitation is a residual hole or defect in the jawbone at the site of an old, or "healed" tooth extraction. Additionally, it will often be present around the apical (end point or tip) area of an infected tooth such as a root canal treated tooth. The contents of a cavitation consist typically of highly toxic, chronically infected, and predominantly necrotic (dead) bone tissue and bone tissue fragments. Under the microscope, the appearance of the contents of a cavitation is essentially the same as that of gangrene seen anywhere else in the body.

It is a fact that cavitations are very commonly found in most people who have had tooth extractions; the vast majority of dental patients have one or more of them. In a review of 112 patients who were explored for possible cavitations, it was found that nearly 90% (313 out of 354) of wisdom tooth extraction sites had cavitated. Many of these cavitations were not at recent extraction sites. Typically, years and often decades had passed since the teeth had been extracted. All of the other extraction sites also demonstrated the ability to cavitate, although the incidence of cavitation lessened as the size of the teeth extracted became smaller or as the amount of infection present at the time of extraction was less. The bigger the hole and more pronounced the infection, the more likely that healing would be incomplete and remain incomplete. Once present, cavitations tend to remain; they will never heal spontaneously. Complete surgical debridement is mandatory. Cavitations do not gradually heal on their own without surgical intervention, no matter how much time is allowed.

Historical Perspectives

Although still not recognized by modern dentistry to be the common and toxic entity that it is, the cavitation was described as far back as 1915 by the dental pioneer, G. V. Black. While Dr. Black did not call what he found a "cavitation," he nevertheless described very accurately the pathology and gross appearance still seen today. Dr. Black considered bone necrosis to be typical of the cavitation lesion and to be the mechanical factor that resulted in the hollowed-out area so often found at the site of an old extraction. The gradual death of bone would result in a softening of the area until it eventually resulted in an actual hole. Dr. Black labeled this process "chronic osteitis," even though he did not completely understand how such extensive internal bone destruction could occur without obvious external signs of inflammation and swelling. He also noted that the patient was not typically acutely ill, and failed to present with symptoms such as fever. Even though Dr. Black realized that the absence of such classical inflammation/infection-associated signs and symptoms flew in the face of standard medical and dental knowledge, he still advocated that such lesions should be thoroughly debrided.

We are now discovering that some disease-causing microorganisms such as mycoplasma do not present with the classic signs and symptoms of infection normally seen on blood tests or clinical evaluation. These "silent" infections often go initially undetected by our standard laboratory tests and can later cause and/or promote the development of diseases such as fibromyalgia, Gulf War Syndrome, and chronic fatigue. Even when such a disease becomes well established, the possibility of occult, or hidden, infection is rarely entertained as a likely cause of the disease or even as a significant contributory factor in its development. Likewise, cavitations are chronically infected and toxic lesions that can also go undetected by standard tests and yet play a substantial role in the initiation and maintenance of chronic disease. Just like in any other area of the body in which gangrene has set in, Dr. Black advocated a thorough surgical debridement of all dead and diseased tissue inside the jawbone. He noted that it was usually easy to enter the thin cap of bone at the old extraction site and then proceed to remove all of the contents and softened, diseased bone until solid bone margins were reached.

Even though Dr. Black was a dental pioneer who is still held in high esteem by dentists today (he is known as the "father of operative dentistry"), his findings on cavitations never were incorporated into current dental thought or dental teaching. There is no way to know whether this omission was deliberate or inadvertent. Regardless of this oversight the appreciation of the existence of cavitations by other dental authors once again emerged in the 1970s. Much of this writing associated cavitations with undiagnosed facial pain syndromes, and the literature began to talk about "NICO," or neuralgia-inducing cavitational osteonecrosis. Neuralgia refers to pain extending along the pathway of one or more nerves. Patients who presented with trigeminal neuralgias and other atypical facial neuralgias were often found to have cavitations at old extraction sites. After the cavitations were properly debrided, many of these patients experienced resolution of their pain.

The scientific literature has also labeled cavitations with several other names. In addition to NICO, they have also been referred to as Ratner, Roberts, or trigger point bone cavities, interference fields, and alveolar cavitational osteopathosis. But regardless of the name, the entity remains the same, although the clinical consequences can vary widely in the afflicted patient.

Diagnosis

As with any other dental or medical condition, the first step in successfully treating a cavitation is to properly diagnosis it. The physician or dentist should take a thorough chronological medical and dental history. The work-up should also include an evaluation of the multiple initiating and predisposing risk factors for the development of a cavitation (see also Appendix III). A comprehensive oral examination should then be performed. Many (but not all) cavitations of the upper jaw can be detected by direct palpation (finger pressure on the bone). Upper jaw cavitations are easier to detect than lower jaw cavitations by palpation due to the differing bone densities of the upper and lower jaws. If the cavitation is near the surface of the bone, pain may be elicited when pressure is applied to the tissue directly overlying the area.

Sometimes cavitations or even root canal treated teeth can cause referred pain to the head and other parts of the body such as the shoulder, hip, or knee. Root canal treated teeth can share this ability with cavitations since the tissue specimen found in the socket of a freshly extracted root canal treated tooth is usually indistinguishable from the contents of a cavitation with regard to toxins, bacteria, and evidence of gangrene. In fact, almost any area of the body can experience referred pain from a cavitation or a root canal treated tooth. Cavitations that produce facial neuralgias form the syndrome called NICO, already mentioned above. However, it is very important to realize that *most* of the time there is *no* associated referred pain with cavitations and root canal treated teeth. Furthermore, when referred pain at some remote site of the body is present, the site of the cavitation itself is frequently pain-free. This referred pain will only resolve after the cavitation has been surgically debrided or the root canal treated tooth has been extracted and the extraction site properly cleaned.

A diagnostic test to determine any link between the area where pain is felt and the cavitation can be performed by injecting a non-vasoconstrictor anesthetic near the site of the cavitation. If the referred pain goes away or is significantly diminished after injection of the local anesthetic, it is probable that the cavitation is the cause of the referred pain. For the reluctant dental surgeon needing justification, surgical treatment of the cavitation is then clearly indicated. Sometimes the referred pain does not go away when local anesthetic is placed near the cavitation. This does not necessarily mean that the cavitation is still not the source of the referred pain. Factors such as decreased blood supply to the bone and lack of adequate access of the anesthesia to the area most responsible for generation of the pain may prevent relief of symptoms. Surgical intervention may still produce positive results. Diagnostic confirmation should always be attempted when referred pain is suspected. Nevertheless, all suspected cavitation sites should be explored and properly debrided if possible, regardless of the presence or absence of associated symptomatology.

As mentioned earlier, it needs to be emphasized that only a small percentage of cavitations produce either local or referred pain. This does *NOT* mean that these cavitations are not producing toxins that may be affecting other parts of the body. The Haley-Pendergrass toxicity test has found *all* cavitation samples tested thus far to be toxic, with most of them proving to be very highly toxic. How these toxins affect an individual will depend upon many factors including genetic susceptibility, immune system function, and the degree of access that the toxins have to the rest of the body. Root canal treated teeth nearly always disseminate their toxins throughout the body and impact health negatively, but a single small cavitation may sometimes have little apparent clinical effect. Conversely, multiple and/or large cavitations in a patient can be the primary reason for a wide variety of advanced degenerative diseases. The bottom line is that all cavitations should be completely debrided, unless some unique clinical circumstance or individual risk/benefit concern indicates otherwise.

X-Raying the Invisible?

The diagnostic tool that has been most used to diagnose cavitations is the panoramic dental x-ray. This large x-ray includes the upper jaw, lower jaw, teeth and sinuses. Sometimes a smaller periapical x-ray that focuses on the root of a tooth or a limited area of the jawbone is used to get a closer view of a particular area. Although many lesions can be seen on a panoramic x-ray, it does not always depict areas of bone in the beginning stages of osteonecrosis, or cavitation formation. Many times these lesions do not show up on x-ray until there is a 50% deterioration of the bone density relative to adjacent normal bone. This is due to the anatomical nature of bone, which is literally a substance comprised of multiple small holes superimposed upon each other and sandwiched between denser outer bone coverings. Remember that an x-ray is a two dimensional picture of a three dimensional object.

These lesions may take on a variety of x-ray appearances. One appearance is a dark space of variable size, indicating a relatively larger hole or space in the bone than is usually present. When a cavitation is surgically explored, it is very common to "fall into" a hole in the bone after very little drilling. The bone surrounding these holes is often very dense with very little blood supply, although the hole itself may have little, and sometimes no bone covering it. Not uncommonly, only a layer of gingiva (gum tissue) covers a cavitation site.

Even though the x-ray remains the tool most commonly used to visualize a cavitation, it is very important to know that an x-ray is generally sub-optimal for this application. Many times a cavitation will not be seen on an x-ray, except by a highly experienced surgeon with an extensive background in working with and diagnosing cavitations. Because they are difficult to consistently image on x-ray, cavitations have been labeled the "invisible osteomyelitis." Practically speaking, what this also means is that an x-ray in which no cavitation is clearly visualized can NEVER be used as the sole reason for concluding that a cavitation is not present. In other words, *a positive x-ray picture can rule IN the presence of a cavitation, but a negative, normal-appearing x-ray picture can never rule OUT the presence of a cavitation.* Even some dentists who are very aware of the presence of cavitations persist in concluding that they cannot be present in a patient who has normal-appearing panoramic dental x-rays. This approach will always miss many more cavitations than it finds. Until a more sophisticated and reliable diagnostic technology is available, old extraction sites must be routinely explored for the presence of cavitations. A short drill line into the jawbone heals very quickly. No damage is done if no cavitation is discovered. Missing a sizeable cavitation is of far more concern than briefly drilling for one and not finding it.

Physical Appearance and Characteristics

The physical appearance of the contents of cavitations can vary widely. Sometimes cavitations are composed of very mushy bone that can contain scattered globules of fat, with an overall likeness to chicken soup without the fat being skimmed.

Cavitation contents may also have a sawdust-like appearance. The contents can even resemble melted chocolate ice cream. Colors described include green, yellow-green, or tarry black. Sometimes the contents are even clear. Consistencies of the contents range from clumps resembling cottage cheese to a loose, runny liquid. Distinctive odors are often present and are invariably unpleasant. Sometimes a sulfurous, "rotten egg" smell is present. Any odor that is associated with tissue breakdown and death secondary to chronic anaerobic bacterial growth and toxicity can occur. Interestingly, the dentist will sometimes miss the smell, but the patient will not. The smell will sometimes literally get inhaled in its entirety by the patient, never reaching the nose of the dentist. Under such circumstances, the patient needs little reassurance that the procedure was necessary.

The degree of development of a cavitation inside the jawbone can vary significantly from one patient to the next. Depending on a number of local and systemic factors, the progressive cellular death of bone tissue as described long ago by Dr. Black can proceed largely unchecked, or it can "stall out" after only a relatively small cavitation has formed. Because of this, the actual configurations of cavitations inside the jawbone vary widely. They can be very focal and virtually impossible to delineate from the adjacent "normal" holes found in non-diseased, cancellous bone. They can also be quite large, in the range of one centimeter in width or even more. Fingerlike projections can evolve, and the overall cavitation can develop an "amoeba-like," amorphous appearance. Sometimes they are rounded and sometimes they are very ragged and irregular along their boundaries. On occasion the boundaries will calcify to a degree, and the ability for such a cavitation to show up on x-ray will be greatly enhanced. When a patient has had consecutive teeth extracted, or is completely edentulous (without teeth), it is very common for cavitations to extend such that interconnections among them are formed. This progresses to the point that some patients who have had all of their teeth extracted will actually have a tubular defect throughout most of their jawbone containing exceptionally large amounts of the toxic cavitation contents. This is referred to as a "channel cavitation." This is also why many patients who have few or no teeth can have as much or more dental toxicity as patients with many remaining teeth. Many edentulous patients are dealing with an enormous amount of toxicity on a daily basis from their extensive cavitation disease.

New Technology

Two new ultrasound computerized imaging instrument have been developed, one already in production and one in development, which are designed specifically to image cavitation lesions of the jawbone. This technology, which is continuing to evolve, may eventually provide the means of reliably detecting the presence and even the three-dimensional structure of cavitations. The efficacy of ultrasound technology has been demonstrated by over 30 years of use in the medical industry. The use of ultrasound is very patient-friendly and considered to be a non-invasive technology, as it uses sound waves instead of radiation to produce an image.

One Ultrasound device, which is already in production, uses a hand-held device (transducer) that emits high frequency sound waves that supposedly pass painlessly through the jawbone and are received on a digitized array. This signal is transferred to the computer monitor after it is converted to a digitally produced 3-D color image that supposedly reflects differences in bone structure and quality. In our opinion, further research must be done to correlate the data generated by the this device with actual clinical presentation and histological study. I [RK] currently do not use an ultrasound imaging device in my diagnosis and treatment planning since to date I have not seen definitive studies proving its efficacy and reproducibility. We hope that someday an accurate and non-invasive diagnostic device will be shown through stringent scientific evaluation to be useful in assisting in the diagnosis of osteonecrotic and osteomyelitic lesions of the jaws. University sponsored studies to evaluate all diagnostic and treatment modalities are needed to further this goal.

A reliable ultrasound technology would not only show the dental surgeon the size, shape, and extent of the cavitation, it could also indicate the type of bone deterioration involved in the lesion. The surgeon would have a much better idea of how to approach the cavitation surgically and how to know when complete debridement was achieved. Currently, cavitation surgery is a procedure guided only by the experience of the surgeon and the "feel" of when diseased bone has been completely evacuated and healthy bone remains. With an established technology, repeat visualizations during the surgery can assure that the debridement is as complete as possible. Furthermore, the use of the ultrasound before surgery can also help determine whether any specific adjunctive treatments, such as the use of bone regeneration or bone replacement therapies, will be indicated at the time of the surgery. And just as significantly, this technology will allow easy and accurate follow-up. Recurrent cavitations would be readily identified, and empiric surgical exploration would no longer need to be done to "make sure" that the worsening of a patient's condition down the road was not due to the recurrence or persistence of one or more cavitations.

Cavitation Frequency

To recognize the scope of this problem, it is absolutely essential to understand how common cavitations are. The routine manner in which dentists extract teeth, including the more extensive surgery involved in removing impacted wisdom teeth, will *ROUTINELY* result in the formation of cavitations. After it became apparent over time that the healing of large molar extraction sites very rarely resulted in the complete filling in of solid, normal bone, it was elected to determine precisely how common cavitation formation was. The statistical incidence of cavitations was first presented in the winter 1996 issue of the *Journal of Advancement in Medicine*. At a dental facility that routinely explored for cavitations at old extraction sites regardless of how normal the x-ray appeared, it was determined that the x-ray was of no help in ruling out the presence of a cavitation. The wisdom teeth extraction sites were found to have cavitated 88% of the time, with the overall incidence of cavitation formation, regardless of site, to be 77%.

As high as this incidence of cavitation formation may seem to be, the real incidence is undoubtedly even higher. Several reasons allow for such a conclusion. In this study, initial cavitation exploration was a blind procedure, and an incorrect angle of drilling could completely miss smaller and oddly-shaped cavitations. Generally, only one initial attempt at drilling into the jawbone was attempted; if the drill burr did not readily fall into a hole, no new drilling angles were attempted. Another factor favoring the underestimation of the true cavitation incidence related to the frequent merging of adjacent cavitations. If one large hole was found at the site of two adjacent extractions, only one cavitation might have been counted. Finally, whenever an area was not explored, it was counted as not having a cavitation. The smaller anterior tooth extraction sites were often not explored when the residual space between the remaining teeth was small. Obviously, small cavitations will always be missed under such circumstances of non-exploration.

There are two very important conclusions that should be reached from this statistical data. One is that cavitations are VERY common. Not a single patient (out of thousands) who had all four wisdom teeth removed was ever found to be cavitations-free. In fact, most had four cavitations, and nearly all the rest had three. The other conclusion is that you should NEVER accept the assurance from your dentist that there is no point in exploring for a cavitation because he or she cannot see one on your dental x-ray. You may be given other reasons for not surgically exploring for a cavitation, and you should discuss these reasons with your dentist so that you are satisfied with that decision. For example, looking for a small cavitation between tightly situated remaining teeth may often not be a reasonable option, but you should not accept that one does not exist because the x-ray does not demonstrate it. And you most definitely cannot accept that a "negative" x-ray is adequate assurance that cavitations have not formed at the extraction sites of larger teeth, as this is almost certainly not the case.

Treatment of Cavitations

Currently, the most effective method of treating cavitations is complete surgical removal of the dead, diseased, and toxin-containing bone. A complete procedure will also include measures to help optimize the patient's ability to grow new, healthy bone which will eventually fill in the cavitation as fully as possible. Too many dental practitioners advocate injecting different substances into the cavitation lesion with the hope of resolving the lesion non-surgically. One increasingly popular substance that is being injected into cavitations and elsewhere in the body is what is known as a Sanum remedy. The Sanum remedies used by dentists are homeopathic in nature, with the hope that so-called "interference fields" and other "blockages" of normal energy flow will be removed or minimized. However, Sanum remedies contain and employ "apathogenic" microorganisms normally found in the body. As we have discussed earlier, both cavitations and root canal treated teeth develop their incredible toxicities because of what happens when the normal, largely apathogenic, microbial flora of the mouth becomes trapped in the oxygen-deprived environments found in these diseased areas of the jawbone. The last thing any clinician should want to do would be to inject any amount of any kind of microorganism into a cavitation, root canal space, or any other area with little or no oxygen and blood supply. This is like throwing gasoline onto the fire. This method of just injecting something into a cavitation and expecting healing will always prove to be ineffective at best and harmful at worst. Once a tissue is dead, it is dead. There are no treatments for gangrene elsewhere in the body except for amputation and removal, or the very life of the patient ends up being threatened.

Even if a Sanum remedy were able to improve the "energy dynamics" of the mouth and body, the body will not be able to clean out a relatively large area of gangrene without a good blood supply, which, by definition, is never present in gangrene. Ultimately, the ultrasound technology being developed will hopefully be effective at stopping the use of this completely non-scientific approach to what is really a straightforward, non-metaphysical problem. Follow-up pictures would consistently demonstrate no improvement and possibly even enlargement of a cavitation after the injection of a Sanum remedy. Placing new microorganisms into a cavitation may well result in a "reactivation" of what had been a gangrenous area that was relatively fixed in size. Also, even when the cavitation is not actually worsened by the Sanum remedy, the patient will lose precious time and money. Ironically, Sanum remedies are quite expensive and a sick patient with cavitations will only remain sick for a longer period and will risk losing hope that this easily addressable condition can be satisfactorily treated.

To re-emphasize, pockets of dead and infected bone have to be surgically debrided, or removed, in order to obtain good healing. Attempting to address "blocked energy flow" with a Sanum remedy should only be considered on lesions or conditions of a non-infective nature. It is never desirable to introduce additional microbes into oxygen-deprived areas of the body. Cleaning out the gangrene from a site in the jawbone is the only proper first step to take in re-establishing a good blood flow to the area. Once an adequate blood supply is established, allowing the immune system and its many components access to the site in need of healing, then healing will occur. No blood, no healing! It is that simple.

If an infected tooth is associated with a cavitation, it is also imperative that it be extracted at the time of cavitation surgery. An infected tooth acts just like a root canal treated tooth in that it can cause or contribute to a cavitation by being a continuing source of bacteria and associated toxins. Such an infected tooth must always be removed before the bone can return to a state of health.

We believe that the surgical protocol for treating the cavitation should utilize proven surgical principles (see also Chapter 8 and Appendix I). Every aspect of the surgical procedure should be based on sound scientific research and established principles documented to promote good healing. To this end, we have spent a great deal of time and energy researching every aspect of this surgical procedure beginning with the methods for diagnosing these cavitation lesions right down to the type of sutures used for closing the surgery site. This is not to say that the protocol that is presented in this book cannot be improved upon. In fact, as new technology and new research becomes available, these treatment procedures will undoubtedly evolve and change to keep up with new findings. However, we believe that this protocol is currently the most effective and we have had very good clinical success in using it to treat our patients.

When the Batteries Die: A Case History

All activity requires energy. This energy can come from many sources, such as the radiation of the sun, the combustion of fossil fuels, the flowing of a river through a dam, or the combining of different chemicals. Energy is just as necessary for running our toaster as it is for powering the space shuttle. Similarly, our bodies also require energy to function. We obtain our energy through the digestion and assimilation of the food that we eat. This food is converted into molecular energy packets, called ATP, by biochemical processes in our bodies. These biochemical processes require enzymes to facilitate this conversion of food to ATP. Without proper enzyme function, the daily needs of life cannot be met. One such enzyme, creatine phosphokinase (CPK), is found in body tissues that have a high demand for the ATP energy packets, as it is essential for maintaining and restoring ATP levels as energy is expended. Not surprisingly, energy-demanding tissues such as muscle and brain require high concentrations of CPK.

It is especially important to understand that the brain has tremendous energy requirements. Functioning of the brain occurs by electrical transmission of impulses in the nerve fibers caused by the intricate transport, release, and uptake of various chemicals called neurotransmitters. All of this activity requires energy. Without ATP to drive the system, the biochemical processes of the brain slow down. The end result is a loss of concentration, an inability to think clearly and a myriad of other seemingly nonspecific symptoms that we commonly label as "brain fog." Just like a portable tape player, which winds down to a slow and barely audible sound when the batteries run low, our brain also slows down when our "ATP batteries" run low. The presence of certain toxins keeps these batteries from ever fully recharging.

The following case history illustrates the significance of energy production in the brain. Cecil, a high-powered business executive, presented to the office with a complex medical history. He had developed multiple chemical sensitivities, poor digestion and bowel function, skin eruptions, and most significantly, psychological problems. All of these symptoms had developed after an extensive dental treatment plan had been executed over a short period of time. He described some of his psychological problems as feeling "not with it" and being "unable to complete thoughts." Sometimes he felt that he could not leave the house because of the inability to cope with the stress of daily interactions with others. Clearly, Cecil was suffering from some form of psychological impairment. But was there a physical, non-psychological reason for his symptoms? His physicians had found no physical cause for his symptoms and felt that they were psychosomatic in nature, finally suggesting to him that he seek counseling.

Intuitively, Cecil knew that something was wrong with his teeth. He began to do his own research and was convinced that his teeth were poisoning him. When Cecil first presented to the office, he expressed a feeling of hopelessness. His clinical examination, including a review of his x-rays, was decidedly unremarkable by traditional dental standards. Often subtle changes in tooth appearance on x-ray such as a slight rounding of the end of the root, poor definition of the canal system in the tooth, and a blending of the tooth image with the surrounding bone indicate a diseased condition. Previous dentists he had seen could find nothing significantly wrong with his teeth or jaw. This is not surprising since most dentists do not consider many of these subtle changes to be clinically significant. For that matter, most dentists were never trained to even recognize many of these subtle changes in the first place. Yet Cecil remained convinced that the root of his problems related back to some infected teeth and cavitations. After careful review of the x-rays and a detailed medical/dental history and dental examination a determination was made that five teeth were infected and required extraction. There was also an area of likely cavitation in the lower left jaw that required surgical cleaning.

The treatment plan was based upon a careful consideration of Cecil's history combined with a more detailed and precise interpretation of his x-ray. Surgical exploration of the cavitation revealed bone that was "mushy" and not well calcified. This "mushiness" was also present in the bone supporting the teeth that were extracted. Such findings should NEVER be present in normal, uninfected teeth. There were also hollow spaces in the bone and areas containing black, necrotic-appearing tissue. Cecil had felt that one of the worst areas in his mouth was in the lower left jaw in the premolar area where two teeth had been previously extracted. He sensed that this area had not been cleaned out properly and had become infected. After this cavitated area was surgically explored and cleaned out, a sample of this diseased bone was sent to a dental pathology laboratory and another sample of this bone was sent for toxicology testing. The pathology reports revealed chronic osteomyelitis, which indicates an ongoing bone infection, and the toxicology testing revealed a very high degree of toxicity as measured by the extent of vital enzyme inhibition. It is interesting to note that CPK, the enzyme that is so critical in energy production in the brain, was inhibited 100%! This means that after exposure to the toxins from the cavitation site, *NO ACTIVE ENZYME REMAINED!* The toxins from the cavitation completely neutralized the CPK that was present. Therefore, when these toxins eventually reach the bloodstream, the lymphatic system, and any other of the body's transport systems, they will also eventually reach the brain and cause inhibition of CPK, with the subsequent loss of energy production. By such a mechanism, the brain's batteries are essentially allowed to "run down." It's no wonder that Cecil was having all of his "psychological" problems.

In 1908, Henry S. Upson, M.D, attending neurologist to Lakeside Hospital in Cleveland, Ohio and a professor of diseases of the nervous system at Western Reserve University, published a book titled *Insomnia and Nerve Strain*. In this book Dr. Upson discusses observed correlations between dental infections and psychiatric disorders. For example, he writes:

> The patient, a young married women twenty-five years of age, rather suddenly developed fearful pain in her head with attacks of hysterical screaming. She began to be very nervous and sleepless, cried easily, and lost weight rapidly.

On the 30th of December an impacted lower third molar was removed. On the 17th of January, 1908, she was better in other ways but the screaming attacks continued. She was given bromides and frequent nourishment. Improvement began on this regimen, and at about this time pain developed in an upper incisor tooth. An abscess was discovered and the tooth removed. *The screaming attacks stopped at once and she has since been perfectly well.* (emphasis added)

There persists today an apathy in the medical and dental professions correlating the significant effects of dental health on systemic health. Interestingly, Dr. Upson also observed the same attitudes in 1908 when he wrote:

> There seems to exist among physicians not only a disregard but a distinct though mild dislike of the teeth as organs to be reckoned with medically, they being as it were an Ishmael, not to be admitted to their pathologic birthright. Ordinary pain at a distance, as headache or neuralgia due to the teeth, though known, is commonly disregarded.

He went on to say:

> Modern psychiatry takes no account of these scattered cases (cases of psychological disorders resolving after elimination of dental infection), and I am not aware that any one has ever looked for dental disease as a cause of insanity, or attempted a cure by its eradication.

Henry A. Cotton also reported on the significance of infection on mental health in the *Journal of Dental Research* as far back as 1919. His article was titled "Oral Infection and Mental Diseases." Why has this incredibly important connection between infection and the mind been so unrecognized and/or ignored? Perhaps you, as the reader, will have to be the one to make this determination. To be sure, it is unlikely that you will currently find a physician correlating mental health with infection from any source, much less infection from the teeth and jawbone. It should also be noted that Cecil showed highly toxic effects on the other five enzymes that were tested along with the CPK. Certainly, it is very reasonable to conclude that these toxins had a wide range of adverse effects on Cecil's health.

Although Cecil has done significantly better since the dental surgery, the implications of his disease and the secondary effects that have resulted need to be fully understood and learned from. Areas in the mouth that would have appeared innocuous to most dentists on clinical and x-ray examination turned out to harbor highly potent toxins that directly and severely impacted on Cecil's health. Unfortunately, Cecil is not the only casualty of dentistry. He is the rule and not the exception, which is the primary reason this book has been written.

Dental Implant Toxicity

A dental implant involves the placement of an anchor material, typically titanium alloy, into the bone at a site where the natural tooth is missing. This anchor material, usually in the form of a screw or cylinder, then allows the placement of a prosthetic tooth, or it can be used to facilitate the retention of a partial or complete denture. The implant is designed to have the bone grow around it and, to a limited degree, into it. Mechanically, a dental implant offers a stability not attainable with partial or permanent dentures since the implant allows a stable anchor into the jawbone, comparable in strength to a healthy tooth root. This solid fixture allows the dentist to place upon it a single prosthetic tooth, a fixed bridge, or an anchor for a partial or a complete denture. As functionality goes, a dental implant is the next best thing to a natural tooth when considering all the types of restorations that are available to the patient. Very similar restorations can be constructed on both implants and natural teeth.

One significant problem with dental implants involves the

type of anchor material typically used. Most implants today are made of titanium alloy, which is the same material that is often used in artificial hips and knees. Although titanium is a fairly biocompatible metal that appears to "get along" with the immune systems of many patients, it is also very brittle. That is why other metals must be added to the titanium to turn it into an alloy that is less susceptible to fracture. These additional metals, as well as the titanium, leach into the body at a low but continual rate. This leaching process must always be kept in mind when determining what treatment is best for the patient.

The material implanted into the jawbone is really only one aspect of the entire dental implant procedure. Since the implant material is only an anchor, a restoration must be placed by attachment to the implant. This creates two additional potential problems:

1. Many restorations are composed of different metals other than titanium alloy, which can produce a dissimilar metal response called galvanism. If proper attention is not paid to the metal used in the dental restoration, the resulting galvanism can actually result in measurable voltages in the mouth, which can further result in a number of undesirable long-term effects on oral and general health.
2. Unlike hip and knee replacements, which are fully enclosed within the body, dental implants are partially placed directly into the bone, while still protruding through the gum tissue into the mouth. Since dental implants are not fully enclosed within the body and protrude through the gum tissue into the mouth, a direct access of bacteria into the bone is facilitated. The gum attachments around implant sites are not the same as the gum attachments around natural teeth. Because of this difference, the gum attachments around the implants are more prone to bacterial invasion when even

the slightest degree of gum inflammation occurs. A direct access of bacteria into the supporting bone can then rapidly occur.

Another problem with dental implants appears to relate directly to the nature of the procedure. The intentional incorporation of a foreign material into an area of growing bone results in some thoroughly predictable responses from the body. The immune system of the patient who undergoes a dental implant will always react to some degree against this insertion of foreign material into the jawbone. This is what the immune system is designed to do. This reaction becomes *auto*immune when metalic ions from the implant combine with normal tissues in the body. While not all patients will show the same reaction to materials implanted within their jawbones, some degree of interaction can always be anticipated. Furthermore, in the patient who is already significantly challenged immunologically from other disease processes, any additional immune challenge, such as that which occurs after the placement of one or more dental implants, may have serious clinical consequences. It should also be realized that the toxicity of most implants extends beyond just an autoimmune reaction.

Probably the most significant reason underlying the toxicity of dental implants has to do with the nature and timing of their insertion. As noted earlier in this chapter, the "ordinary" way in which dentists continue to perform tooth extractions assures a very high incidence of cavitation formation at those sites, especially when involving the larger teeth. A cavitation not only harbors toxic microorganisms and their highly toxic metabolites, it also is the last place in the body where good healing will ever be seen, in the absence of thorough surgical debridement. However, the very existence of cavitations and their toxicity is still largely unknown to most dentists and dental sub-specialists. Because of this, the average dentist proceeding to insert a dental implant into the jawbone views the relatively recent extraction site as a good place for getting the implant material well-situated prior to the anticipated healing-in of bone there. But as we now know, choosing this implant site means that a foreign material is actually being screwed or tapped into an area of potential, and likely active, cavitation formation. This assures that bacteria and their toxins are intimately involved in what should be a sterile and non-toxic healing process. Furthermore, the very insertion of the metal implant further introduces these bacteria and bacterial toxins deeper into areas of the jawbone that had not yet been infected or that were not already dying from the cavitation process.

What to do? Well, for all of the reasons mentioned above, the dental implant procedure should generally be avoided entirely if at all possible. However, if unique mechanical and dental considerations strongly indicate the need for a dental implant, or if conventional complete or partial dentures have significant contraindications, then the dental implant might be considered a possible alternative. We say "might" since some degree of autoimmune response can always be anticipated after the implant procedure.

How should an implant be performed in order to minimize the chances of worsening the patient's general medical condition? Very simply, the least toxic implant material should be used and only placed in an area of healthy bone already healed or in the process of healing. As a general rule, titanium looks to be a very promising material with good mechanical qualities and a relatively low toxicity profile. Both the primary and secondary implant materials, as well as the other materials involved in finishing the implant procedure, should be chosen based on least reactive immune serum biocompatibility profiling (see Appendix V).

Once all of the best materials have been chosen, it is very important to be sure that no cavitation is present at the site of planned implant insertion. Even if the extraction was performed in an optimal fashion and the site was thoroughly debrided of all necrotic and infected bone at the time of the procedure, the lack of subsequent cavitation formation is never fully assured. As discussed earlier, many different factors promote the formation of a cavitation. An incomplete cleaning of the bony socket after a tooth extraction is only one of them. Practically speaking, then, an implant should never be performed at an old extraction site until surgical exploration confirms that an infected, toxic defect has not developed at that site.

The true toxicity of such an optimally placed dental implant is unknown. We have seen multiple patients show striking clinical improvement after the removal of one or more dental implants, much like we have seen with the removal of root canal treated teeth and with the debridement of cavitations. However, the placement of a dental implant using a metal such as titanium alloy into an area of healthy bone without cavitation has not been investigated fully enough to know how much or how little toxicity will result. The autoimmune reaction alone, without associated infection and toxicity from inducing further cavitation formation deep at the implant site, could be of relatively minor significance in the well-chosen patient. Yet, there still could be some patients for which the autoimmune reaction alone even after an optimally performed implant would nevertheless be of significant clinical consequence.

One other consideration to keep in mind before proceeding with even an optimally performed dental implant has to do with the amount of bone volume required in the implant procedure. Unlike most other dental procedures, dental implants require a substantial degree of thickness of the jawbone for their placement. As long as the procedure is permanent, and the implant is well integrated and never removed, this is of little consequence. However, the removal of dental implants may result in significant bony defects and loss of bone. Complete healing and filling-in of bone may never occur. In some patients, the subsequent placement of good-fitting dentures can be significantly impaired by such a loss of bone. Furthermore, subsequent trauma or infection can also make jaw fracture a greater future risk at sites where the jawbone structure has been weakened in this way.

8

PROPER PRE-OPERATIVE AND POST-OPERATIVE CARE

Overview

The introduction of antibiotics in medicine revolutionized the treatment of many diseases. The appropriate dispensing of antibiotics has saved many lives, but they should not be prescribed indiscriminately or without due consideration of potential side effects, such as the development of more tenacious, antibiotic-resistant bacterial strains. Antibiotics have been routinely overused for a long time now, and many types of bacteria have since developed into new strains that are resistant to the same antibiotics that were once effective against them. This has resulted in the development of newer and even more potent antibiotics that are often much less specific in the bacteria that they attack.

The destruction of the "good" bacteria as well as the disease-producing ones will often result in a new set of clinical problems for the patient. Other microorganisms, such as yeasts, can take hold in the absence of the bacteria that should be present. Once such new and toxic microorganisms have set up housekeeping in the body, their elimination typically requires more antimicrobial therapy, since stopping the initial antibiotic therapy is often not enough to restore the proper balance of good bacteria in the body. The new drugs will often result in further superinfection with other more dangerous microbes that would never have gotten a foothold inside the normal body without the initial antibiotic intervention. More is not always better, since the cure can sometimes be worse than the disease. So what to do?

Weighing Risk Versus Benefit

In determining whether or not to use antibiotics as a protective measure when performing a medical procedure, it is important to examine the risks of not administering them versus the possible side effects that might occur from administering them. Remember that the toxic overgrowth of harmful microbes after antibiotic therapy occurs more often when one or more of the following conditions exist:

1. Very prolonged usage (weeks to months or LONGER)
2. High dosages
3. Combination therapy with multiple antibiotics
4. Combination therapy with antibiotics and other antimicrobial agents, such as anti-fungal agents
5. Repeated courses of therapy for a recurrent or chronic condition
6. Inappropriate prescription (antibiotics for a viral infection rather than a bacterial infection)
7. Using the most potent antibiotic at the outset
8. Addressing and treating only the symptomatology rather than the cause of an infection-related condition

In spite of the conditions noted in the above list, antibiotic therapy still can play a significant role in the achievement of safe dental surgery. The scientific literature clearly shows that oral pathogens can easily relocate elsewhere in the body, and the toxins they produce can also disseminate from the mouth, as well as be produced at a site of new microbial growth elsewhere in the body. The literature also reveals that these oral pathogens with their associated toxins can become especially entrenched in the bone, causing a condition called osteomyelitis. Dental surgery will typically also involve jawbone surgery, and the dental surgeon must be especially careful not to initiate or promote a chronic osteomyelitis condition in the jawbone. It would therefore appear that the *judicious* use of an appropriate combination of oral and intravenous antibiotics should be included in the standard protocol for cavitation surgery and for the extraction of root canal treated teeth.

Just as orthopedic surgeons are highly concerned with infection when operating on bone elsewhere in the body and use the strictest of aseptic techniques, dental surgeons should exert an even *higher* degree of concern and caution. The mouth is literally teeming with a wide variety of microorganisms including bacteria, fungi, protozoa, and multiple other species of microbes, yet the body is often given little support in initiating a non-contaminated start to healing after the completion of many dental surgeries. At the very least, the oral surgeon should follow *all* of the precautions employed by the orthopedic surgeons. To be sure, orthopedic surgeons would employ even more exacting precautions if their surgical environments contained the microbes found in the mouth.

Oral Pathogens and Systemic Effects

More than 400 bacterial species have been found in the oral cavity as well as fungi, mycoplasma species, mycetes, protozoa, and viruses. These organisms can easily gain access to the bloodstream, fascial planes (the spaces between adjacent tissues), bony cavities, lymphatic system, nerves, mucous membrane tissues, and the respiratory and gastrointestinal tracts. Both inhalation and swallowing, which are continuous activities, promote the dissemination of the mouth's microorganisms. The systemic spread of bacteria, bacterial toxins, and the resulting immune complexes throughout the human body can result in a wide variety of diseases. Tiny amounts of bacteria will often find their way into the blood, only to be thwarted and eliminated by a competent immune system.

Larger numbers of bacteria, such as can arise from an infected site in the mouth, will typically overwhelm the protective capacities of the immune system and eventually establish a secondary site of infection elsewhere in the body, or at least result in the body-wide spread of un-neutralized toxins from the original infection site. Antibiotics can help to prevent the occurrence of a secondary infection after oral surgery, which can sometimes cause the release of a very large bacterial challenge into the bloodstream. Of course, antibiotics will have no effect on toxins that have already been produced and released.

Practical Prevention and Protection

Recent scientific research has revalidated the fact that oral microbes can enter the bloodstream and cause focal infections in tissues in distant parts of the body. Extractions and other surgical procedures, such as cavitation surgery, are major, traumatic dental manipulations. They can facilitate the direct entrance into the bloodstream of the microbes that are present in the oral cavity, as well as the microbes and toxins that are already present in the infected teeth, or other operative sites.

It is therefore advisable to utilize a protocol that will:

1. Reduce the level of toxic oral microbes in the mouth as

much as possible prior to surgical procedures.
2. Reduce the level of toxic microbes in the infected tissue targeted for surgery.
3. Destroy the toxic microbes that do gain access to the bloodstream during the surgical procedure, and minimize the possibility that a focal infection will develop remotely from the mouth.

Reducing Oral Microbes

It is important for the teeth, tongue, gums, and entire oral cavity to be as clean as possible before planning any oral surgery. If there is plaque or calculus build-up on the teeth, they should be cleaned by a dental hygienist at least a few days to a few weeks before the surgery. The patient needs to pay especially close attention to oral hygiene for at least one to two weeks preceding the appointment. This attention includes:

1. Brushing thoroughly and *properly* three or more times per day. Consider using an electric toothbrush.
2. Flossing thoroughly and *properly* one or more times per day.
3. Using an oral water irrigating device.
4. Using a tongue scraper if it is difficult to keep the tongue clean.
5. Using an oral antimicrobial rinse that does not contain alcohol or fluoride. The Dental Herb Company's all natural toothpaste, rinse, and concentrate works well.
6. For three days prior to surgery and for two weeks after surgery, chlorhexidine gluconate 0.12% (available by prescription) anti-microbial rinse should be used three times a day.

Immediately preceding the surgery, the patient should cleanse the oral cavity well and rinse thoroughly with chlorhexidine gluconate 0.12%. Prior to beginning the surgical procedure, the surgeon should laser the sulcus (tooth-gum margin area) of the tooth to be removed or adjacent to the areas being prepared for surgery. Appropriate soft tissue laser curettage will significantly reduce the bacterial count. During the entire surgical procedure, the surgical site should be flushed with generous amounts of sterile saline solution to continuously remove bacteria and debris from the surgical site. Plain water should never be used to irrigate the bone, and although Betadine and hydrogen peroxide are well known anti-microbial agents, they should not be placed into the surgical site. These can inhibit the formation of new bone, as can some antibiotics if they are placed topically in the surgical site.

Antibiotic Administration

One suggested protocol would include the following: During surgery, a mixture of IV antibiotics containing vancomycin and clindamycin should be administered. This combination provides the most broad-spectrum coverage against the organisms found in the oral cavity and especially those that can cause osteomyelitis. Oral clindamycin should be administered the day before surgery and for three days after surgery. If a patient cannot take these antibiotics, intravenous Unasyn in conjunction with oral Augmentin is the alternate antibiotic treatment regimen of choice.

Protecting the Gut

Probiotics, a commercial preparation that is a source of "friendly" gut bacteria, should be taken before, during, and after the time period that antibiotics are administered. This can help prevent the development of yeast infections and the resultant diarrhea and/or vaginitis that sometimes occurs when too many of the "friendly" bacteria are killed by antibiotics.

When antibiotics are being administered, it is best to take the probiotics at least one hour after taking the antibiotics. Avoid taking them together at the same time during the day.

Other Protective Measures

To supplement the action of antibiotics, other methods of protecting the body from systemic damage that can result from the invasion of oral pathogens may also be utilized. This includes taking an extract of olive leaf, or any of several other "natural" anti-microbial products for several days preceding and following surgery. Skin contact infrared therapy, which has an antibacterial and antiviral effect, can also be utilized. In addition, oxidative therapy, such as the intravenous infusion of dilute hydrogen peroxide, is another highly effective adjunctive treatment.

Liberal use of vitamin C is also critical in minimizing the clinical impact from the acute release of bacterial toxins and in lessening the likelihood of effective bacterial spread to remote sites. When possible, an infusion of 50 or more grams of vitamin C, as a sodium ascorbate solution in sterile water, should be administered before, during, and after the dental procedure. Depending upon the clinical situation, one or more additional infusions may be administered in the immediate preoperative days. Liberal doses of oral vitamin C should also be taken after the procedure. Individual dosing will vary, but *grams* of vitamin C will always be the indicated dosing, not *milligrams*, during this critical period of healing and recovery. Typical total daily oral doses of vitamin C will range from 5 to 15 grams. This total dose is best taken in three or more divided doses during the day. If there are any concerns that healing and the clinical postoperative status of the patient are sub-optimal, the vitamin C infusions should be continued. An optimal hydration status must also be maintained, with a minimum intake of two quarts of purified water per day.

Unipolar Magnetic Therapy

Magnetic therapy has been coming into vogue of late. Athletes use magnetic applications to their limbs and joints for pain relief. Many different magnetic devices and applications are now beginning to appear. However, magnetic therapy is a double-edged sword, as are most effective therapies, and it must be employed under the guidance of someone having a proper understanding of how magnetics promote healing.

Good bio-magnets have clearly marked north and south poles. *ONLY* the north pole should ever be applied against the body! Furthermore, some magnetic companies can have opposite definitions of the two poles. They arbitrarily label one pole north and one pole south. The Magnetizer company, listed in the Resources section at the end of the book, labels the north pole green and the south pole red (see Appendix V). A good magnetometer can help you figure out the proper polar orientation of magnets that are not clearly and properly labeled.

Applying the north pole of a strong bio-magnet against inflamed and/or infected tissue, in both the mouth and elsewhere, is enormously effective in accelerating the healing process. Quite often, the prompt application of such magnets over the cheek against extraction sites can completely prevent *any* postoperative pain after the local anesthesia has worn off! Furthermore, the north pole inhibits the growth of microorganisms, which is also very important in supporting the healing process. Finally, unipolar magnetic therapy promotes the regrowth of bone at extraction and cavitation sites, which makes recurrent disease much less likely to occur. The opposite (south) side of the magnet will impair good healing in the mouth as effectively as the north pole will support good healing there. If you are not sure which pole is being applied to your cheek, or any other part of your body, don't use that magnet.

Summary

One of the major goals of cavitation surgery or extraction of root canal treated teeth is to eliminate a focus of infection and/or toxicity from the body. The surgery cannot be considered a success if it results in a systemic infection or a focal infection in another area of the body due to the translocation of oral microorganisms or pathogens from the surgical site. One problem has been exchanged for another. Even if the cavitation debridement or the root canal extraction is a technical success, the ultimate goal of the surgery, the long-term health of the patient, will not have been given its best chance to be realized. The choice of effective antibiotics, along with their prudent use, can greatly assist in attaining the goals of involved oral surgery and in protecting the patient from local as well as systemic infection. Laser treatment of the gums will kill many of the bacteria present in the spaces between the gum and the tooth, and the risk of infection after surgery will be further reduced. It is highly recommended to use this procedure preoperatively in conjunction with the prudent utilization of antibiotic therapy.

9

PERIODONTAL DISEASE

Overview

Periodontal disease literally refers to disease occurring around the tooth. In this chapter we will explore a description of periodontal disease as well as the mechanisms in which periodontal disease progresses to affect local as well as systemic sites throughout the body.

Commonly, periodontal disease primarily involves variable degrees of gingival, or gum, inflammation and bone destruction. Advanced periodontal disease can proceed deep into the space between the tooth and the gum tissue (called the periodontal sulcus), eventually leading to tooth loss due to chronic infection along with the actual loss of bone forming the tooth socket. Based on the information that has already been covered in this book, it should be apparent that any condition that harbors infection deep in the gum tissue or in the tooth socket will result in the production of anaerobic bacterial toxins just as is seen with root canal treated teeth and cavitations. What may be less apparent is the significant negative consequence of mild to moderate gum disease that has not yet progressed deeply into the tooth and tooth socket.

To briefly recap some important concepts, many of the bacteria normally found in the mouth become little toxin-producing factories when their normal oxygen supply is eliminated or severely reduced. This oxygen deprivation is known as the anaerobic or near-anaerobic state. When this oxygen supply is lacking, the bacteria change their metabolism and start producing different metabolic by-products that turn out to be enormously potent toxins. Similarly, this is essentially what happens in root canal treated teeth and cavitations. The bacteria (potentially over 400 different species) are trapped without oxygen, and toxins continue to be produced.

The same reasoning applies to periodontal disease affecting only the upper gum surfaces at the area of contact with the tooth. Normally, there is a fluid flow from the inside of the tooth outward that proceeds between the tooth surface and the gum. Fluid normally flows from the inside of this space into the mouth. This normal state of fluid flow helps the tooth-gum area to keep itself "flushed-out" and relatively free of bacteria and other factors that would promote inflammation and eventual infection of the tooth and/or gums. In root canal treated teeth, however, the tooth pulp has been removed and this important natural fluid flow is lacking. Therefore, any bacteria that are present in the gingival sulcus (the space between the upper gum and the crown of the tooth) can readily make their way into the porous dentin tubules. This not only infects the tooth but also serves as a reservoir for re-infection of the gum tissue in the event that the initial gum infection manages to resolve. And even though the root of the tooth is covered with an outer layer called cementum, which is impervious to bacterial invasion, this layer is usually removed during routine teeth cleaning, thereby making the dentin tubules more prone to bacterial invasion. The normal fluid flow found in vital healthy teeth is important in keeping them uninfected. And the loss of this fluid flow is just one more factor working to keep root canal treated teeth infected. Also, the gums above root canal treated teeth remain infected more readily due to the ever present and nearby bacterial reservoir below them.

Proliferation of bacteria and the presence of other pathogenic, disease-causing organisms can lead to the first stage of gum disease called *gingivitis*. Gingivitis is characterized by mild inflammation of the gum tissue. Poor nutrition and poor local dental hygiene are important reasons why these microbes can initiate gingivitis. This inflammation, if left unchecked, can then progress to *periodontitis* with the presence of not only a greater number of microbes, but also more pathogenic bacteria. Advanced gum disease can also show the presence of relatively large microorganisms such as amoeba. The continued progression of advanced periodontal disease causes a breakdown of the bone socket, eventually resulting in tooth loss.

Once gum inflammation becomes established, the same conditions for anaerobic bacterial metabolism as are seen in root canal treated teeth and cavitations exist. Not surprisingly, then, many of the same toxins are produced as well. Periodontal disease, if present throughout the mouth, can produce as much and even more collective toxicity than one or more root canal treated teeth and cavitations. Incredibly, the surface area of the tooth-gum interface around all of the teeth equals the surface area of the underside of your arm! This large surface area is a significant factor in enabling the production of greater numbers of anaerobic bacterial toxins. In one sense, widespread periodontal disease is very much like having a root canal treated tooth and/or cavitation at every tooth site.

Clinical Consequences of Periodontal Disease

Multiple scientific articles have clearly established that periodontal disease is associated with an increased risk of heart attack (also see Appendix II). This should come as no surprise when one realizes that chronically inflamed and infected gums not only produce toxins that end up circulating throughout the body, they also provide a fairly continuous seeding of bacteria and other toxin-producing microbes throughout the body as well. Both the microbes and the toxins place a great deal of chronic stress on the body and the immune system, and heart disease is one of the direct consequences of this stress.

Let's look more closely at just one aspect of the systemic effects of periodontal disease that has been under recent investigation. This aspect is the link between periodontal disease and increased risk of heart attack and stroke.

What is the possible mechanism of action in this link? As the pathogenic bacteria build up in the spaces between the teeth and gums, the body activates the immune system to try to fight this infection. It is important to remember that periodontal disease is an infection, just like any other infection in the body. However, the infection present in periodontal disease (and likewise in root canal treated teeth and cavitations) can contain any of approximately 400 different species of bacteria, as noted earlier.

The body attempts to fight this infection by sending in white blood cells. These are some of the important cells of the immune system that fight disease. However, to gain access into the infected periodontal space, or sulcus, these white blood cells have to migrate outside of the blood stream to eventually enter this dental area. In order to do this, blood vessels in the gum tissue must become "leaky" to allow passage of the white blood cells into the sulcus. This is accomplished by producing inflammation, which is at least partially caused when specific immune cells release chemicals called cytokines. Certain cytokines promote inflammation and facilitate this passage of white blood cells into the sulcus to fight the periodontal infection. An example of such gingival disease is seen with bleeding gums, which is a reliable indicator that an inflammatory process is present and is caused by some degree of infection in the gums.

When inflammation is present in the gums allowing the passage of the white blood cells into the tissue, it also allows bacteria to move in the *opposite* direction, eventually reaching the bloodstream. These bacteria and their toxins can initiate processes that eventually result in the actual damage of the inside smooth lining of the blood vessel walls. Cytokines produced by the white blood cells in response to injury or infection promote inflammation and initiate the "up-regulation" of oxidized cholesterol into specific white blood cells called macrophages. After the damage has been initiated, cholesterol and other blood fats can be deposited at these injured and infected sites by the macrophages in an effort to repair the damage to the blood vessel wall. This repair process would work perfectly well and most likely would not lead to arteriosclerosis, or arterial narrowing and blockages, if the initiating factors were temporary and not continuous. However, periodontal disease, along with all of the other dental infections, continues to supply an onslaught of microbes and toxins. Because of this, the very mechanism that would heal the blood vessel gets chronically over stimulated, and the very healing response itself is largely what ultimately narrows and blocks off blood vessels. *Acute* inflammation is very important in the initiation of healing. However, *chronic* inflammation is the worst enemy of good healing. As the inflammatory/infective/toxic process continues, the build-up of repair cells and cholesterol grows and continues to narrow the artery.

In the blood vessel wall, this repair process can be highly unstable due to inflammation and infection at the site of repair. Such a site is called an unstable plaque. In fact, many heart attacks are caused by the breakup of such "hot" plaques, which can precipitate the sudden, total blockage of a coronary (heart) artery, rather than by the more gradual narrowing of a coronary artery by larger, more stable plaques.

To make matters worse, the presence of bacteria found in these arterial narrowing can help to initiate the clumping and sticking together of platelets. The sticking together of platelets often starts the blood clotting process. By introducing bacteria into the bloodstream that make platelets clump together, we have the potential for a heart attack or stroke. At least one species of bacteria commonly found in the mouth, *Streptococcus sanguis*, is known to help cause platelets to stick together. This is a species of bacteria that is also known to cause heart infections, or bacterial endocarditis.

Although this dental infection/heart disease correlation has been reported in the literature primarily for periodontal disease, it can also be correlated to root canal treated teeth and cavitations.

Any infection in the body can also result in the development of acute and chronic autoimmune reactions against different body tissues. Gum infections are no exception. An autoimmune reaction occurs when the immune system attacks native tissues and cells that have been altered slightly by the infection or toxin so that the immune system no longer recognizes it as native. Instead, it views parts of the body that it should be protecting from disease as being foreign and needing to be attacked and neutralized, rather than protected.

Also, some bacteria can masquerade themselves in such a fashion that the immune system disregards them as normal body tissue. Called "bacterial mimicry," this is an attempt by the bacteria to avoid recognition and destruction by the immune system. There is often some degree of autoimmune reaction underlying many infections that are not typically recognized as autoimmune diseases. It is important to realize that many autoimmune diseases are actually infectious in origin. The infective form of autoimmune disease is far more common than the incidence of some of the well-known autoimmune diseases such as lupus or scleroderma. However, even the well-known autoimmune diseases can also often have an infectious origin and/or a contributing factor that is infectious in nature.

It is nearly impossible to maintain healthy gums when one is a smoker. Smoking neutralizes an enormous amount of vitamin C in the body, and this vitamin C depletion greatly facilitates gum infection. In fact, biopsy studies have shown that inflamed and infected gum tissue is quite low in its tissue vitamin C levels. Furthering this vicious cycle is that the gum infections and associated toxins can more readily build up in a body with ever-decreasing vitamin C levels. This vitamin C depletion further lessens the immune protection against the progression of the gum disease and its associated toxin production.

Treating and Preventing Periodontal Disease

A good program of proper nutrition and proper supplementation is extremely important in the maintenance of good gum health as well as general body health. Local gum care is important, but good nutrition and supplementation cannot be minimized or neglected, even if the local gum care is meticulous. Optimal nutrition is an extensive subject that will not be addressed here, but the reader is directed to the Resources section at the end of this book for direction to reliable information on this important subject (see Appendix V).

Dental water irrigation devices should be utilized regularly. Water with hydrogen peroxide is a good tooth and gum irrigant. Peroxide releases oxygen that kills the bacteria that live deep within the periodontal space. These anaerobic bacteria can be readily killed by the release of oxygen from the peroxide.

Proper tooth brushing with a fluoride-free toothpaste or other dentifrice is important. Fluoride-containing toothpastes should be not be used since fluoride is another cumulative toxin that should be avoided as much as possible. Tooth brushing should be accompanied by the direct removal of the daily accumulation of food debris with careful, non-traumatic flossing. This practice can reduce plaque formation and lessen the likelihood of developing periodontal disease.

Summary
1. Periodontal disease is an infection.
2. This infective process can lead to not only local problems such as tooth loss, but also the proliferation of bacteria and the production of bacterial toxins. These microbes and their toxins can spread throughout the body, and the body's own immune response to this infectious and toxic presence can have serious systemic consequences such as heart attack or stroke. Many other systemic diseases, such as chronic fatigue syndrome, may also have their origin in, or a significant contribution from, sites of oral infection.
3. The elimination of active periodontal disease involves elimination of the bacteria that cause the disease. Therapies such as regular cleanings that remove the bacterial plaque deep within the sulcus, as well as periodontal laser treatments to kill the bacteria in the sulcus, are important effective ways to treat periodontal disease. Sometimes antibiotics must be used and occasionally periodontal surgery must be performed to eliminate and heal deep periodontal pockets, which then allows for effective home care to maintain optimal gum health.
4. And, of course, all root canal treated teeth must be removed since they are a reservoir for bacteria and bacterial toxins, and can re-infect the gums propagating periodontal disease.

10

FREQUENTLY ASKED QUESTIONS

What is a root canal procedure and why is it performed?
First, let's look at the anatomy of a tooth. The part of the tooth that is visible when looking in the mouth is called the crown of the tooth. What you do not see are the roots of the tooth. The roots extend into the jawbone and anchor the tooth to the bone.

Upon viewing an extracted tooth, many people are surprised at how long the roots can be. Front teeth generally have only one root while molars (back teeth) generally have two or three roots. Furthermore, the inside of a root has a canal that is much less dense than the rest of the tooth, containing nerves and blood vessels. This canal runs from the end tip of the root up to an even larger hollowed-out area in the crown of the tooth, much like the configuration of a single-scoop ice cream cone. This entire hollowed-out area is called the pulp chamber. The complex of associated nerves and blood vessels in this pulp chamber is called the root canal system.

As the purpose of the root canal system is to supply nerves and blood vessels to the tooth, the root canal system is literally filled from tip to crown with nerve tissue, connective tissue, and blood vessels. A root canal procedure is generally performed when this pulp tissue inside the tooth becomes infected and painful. This can occur because of an earlier trauma to the tooth, as can happen when something hard is bitten upon with too great a force. Tooth decay may extend completely through the crown and result in a chronic infection in the pulp chamber. This infection will eventually cause the death of much of the tissue in the root canal system. However, enough of the nerve supply to the tooth may remain resulting in significant chronic pain from the infected tooth. The infection spreads down the root and into the surrounding bone and dentin tubules, after which the complete eradication of the infecting microbes is impossible to achieve.

Although pain can be present at any time during this infective process, the infection can sometimes spread into the surrounding bone without any pain. The goal of the root canal procedure is to remove much of the infected and necrotic (dead) tissues in the root canal system, and then seal the entire root canal system with a rubber-like material called gutta-percha combined with a paste sealer. This will usually result in relief of the associated tooth pain, which is the primary clinical goal of the root canal procedure. However, the infection remains until the tooth is extracted and the socket thoroughly cleaned out.

Does a root canal procedure remove all of the infection from the tooth?

No. There are several reasons that you cannot sterilize an infected tooth. The first reason is that along with the main canal that runs the entire length of the root, there are additional, much smaller, canals that extend away from the main canal at varying angles to the exterior of the root. It is impossible to clean these canals with root canal instruments because the instruments can only reach the main canal. Also, many of the roots are curved or have points of branching within the main canal system, making even it impossible to clean in its entirety.

Most pathology reports from extracted root canal treated teeth report necrotic debris (dead tissue remnants) remaining in the primary root canal. That means that even the main canal was not entirely cleaned and sealed. This is seen with straight as well as curved roots. It is seen in teeth treated by root canal specialists as well as by general dentists.

Finally, and perhaps most important, the body of the tooth surrounding the main canal is *not* solid. Except for the enamel on the exterior of the tooth, the entire tooth is composed of a material called dentin. Dentin is porous like a sponge. It contains an extensive maze of very tiny dentin tubules that run from the nerve canal out towards the exterior of the tooth. However, these tubules do not always travel in a straight line. Instead, they form a complex interconnecting network within the entire tooth. It is estimated that if you were to take the tubules from the relatively small front tooth and put them end-to-end, they would stretch for three miles! Now, a front tooth has only one root. Molars can have two or more roots. Bacteria can fit up to three across in these tubules. So you can imagine how many bacteria can live in an infected tooth. No root canal procedure can ever reach and clean out bacteria and other microbes that have already reached this system of dentin tubules. Furthermore, once the pulp gets infected, the dentin tubules will always be infected as well. This is the primary flaw with the root canal procedure: Pain may be eliminated but the infection will always remain. Clinically, the tooth can feel fine while remaining infected and highly toxic.

Isn't there anything that can be used to sterilize the bacteria in these dentin tubules?

Currently, nothing is available that can sterilize the intricate lattice of dentin tubules of their microbial invaders once they have settled in. In fact, Dr. Weston Price, who performed the defining work on the pathology of root canals, attempted to sterilize the tubules by using potent antibacterial solutions applied to the inside canals of *extracted* teeth. He used very strong chemicals-chemicals that would be too toxic to actually use inside the mouth of a patient. Yet, he was still unable to sterilize the infected dentin tubules. The intricate network of tubules does not allow perfusion of irrigating solutions. Furthermore, the removal of most of the nerve and blood supply in the pulp chamber also keeps the patient's immune system cells from having the necessary access to the dentin tubules required to cause a natural sterilization of this area. Healing anywhere in the body requires a good blood supply or it will not occur; infection will always persist under such circumstances.

Why can't a laser sterilize the tubules?

By definition, laser light is effectively "gathered" and focused to travel in a very straight line. In fact, it is this characteristic of a laser that distinguishes it from an ordinary light source, however intense that light may be. Since the laser is pointing down into the canal of the tooth, the laser energy travels straight down the root and cannot reach any lateral, offshoot areas of the tooth that take off at various angles from the primary direction of the laser. Therefore, although the laser may be useful in helping to sterilize most of the main canal, it cannot sterilize the lateral canals or the dentin tubules that may be at right angles from the targeted path of the laser.

In an attempt to see if the dentin tubules on an extracted

tooth could be sterilized with a laser, the root canal system of this extracted tooth was cleaned and enlarged in the same way a root canal would be performed on a tooth still in the mouth. A sample of bacteria was then taken from beneath the gum around a tooth in the mouth. This sample contained live bacteria. The sample was then placed in a groove prepared on the side of the root. The laser was then focused into the root canal of the tooth at a power setting and time of exposure that would be far above what could be safely tolerated during an actual root canal procedure in the mouth. The bacteria sample was removed from the side of the tooth and placed under a microscope. The bacteria were all very much alive. We do not believe that the laser can effectively sterilize the dentin tubules, no matter how skilled the dentist may be at using this device. Any bacteria that are not the direct path of the laser will simply not be killed.

Many clinicians note that when a laser is shining inside a tooth, the whole tooth seems to "light up." This does mean that some of the light is scattering throughout the tooth. However, this scattered light has none of the effects of the primary lased light. Such scattered light cannot kill bacteria. Rather, this is simply ordinary light that trans-illuminates and nothing more.

I heard that there is a material called Biocalex that is supposed to penetrate the dentin tubules and kill bacteria. Would this be an option for effective sterilization of root canals?

We do not believe that the Biocalex brand of root canal filling material, or any other root canal filling material developed to date, can ever achieve the goal of a sterile, non-toxic root canal treated tooth. A tooth that was treated with Biocalex was tested for the degree of toxicity as measured by enzyme inhibition of several important human enzymes. This tooth tested "extreme" on all the enzymes tested, indicating a high level of toxicity from the products of bacterial metabolism inside the tooth.

No root canal filling material can completely fill the miles of infected dentin tubules found in all root canal treated teeth. Biocalex may fill the core area of the canal a bit better than other filling materials such as gutta-percha, but it cannot fill all the dentin tubules. Clinically speaking, even a slight decrease in the toxic content of an infected tooth is really irrelevant, since the remaining toxins are still overwhelmingly toxic. 80 to 90% of the toxins in a typical root canal treated tooth are just as clinically devastating as 100% of the toxins. Biocalex should never be used with the excuse that a "less toxic" root canal results. 90% of an atomic bomb will blow you away just as effectively as 100% of the blast.

What about ozone treatment?

Ozone may be effective in killing bacteria within the root canal system but we do not believe that it kills bacteria within the dentin tubules. Just as with other agents, ozone simply cannot penetrate the entire system of dentin tubules.

Some people claim to heal cavitations with ozone without the need for surgery. Although we think that ozone can be an important adjunctive treatment that helps to promote good healing, nothing can turn dead bone into live bone. If a cavitation is lacking a blood supply and the surrounding bone is infected, surgery must be performed to remove the dead and infected bone and to establish a blood supply to the area. Ozone or other remedies that are often injected into cavitation sites can never substitute for the healing effect that occurs when dead and infected bone and tissue is removed. When gangrene occurs, the affected tissue must be amputated or otherwise removed, no matter where it is in the body.

Why not just take out the root canal and leave the tooth?

This is a question that we often hear. The fact is that the root canal procedure has to be performed within the tooth. The only way to take out the root canal is to take out the tooth entirely.

How do I know if this root canal treated tooth is affecting my health? Will my physical ailments get better if I extract root canal treated teeth and I have cavitations cleaned out?

Cause-and-effect is often difficult to establish in as complex a biological system as the human body. We, along with other scientists and clinicians, believe that many diseases are infectious and toxic in origin. However, most diseases are aggravated or prevented from resolving by multiple other factors. The overall physical and psychological health of the patient, coupled with environmental exposures and genetic predisposition, all play a role in the disease process. We feel that by unloading the body of a known and severe biological toxic stressor such as a root canal treated tooth or a cavitation, we are eliminating a possible cause of a person's disease. At the very least, the immune system becomes less burdened and capable of better protecting against other infectious pathogens. Furthermore, the unburdening of the immune system allows it to be stronger in general and more effective in protecting against other seemingly unrelated diseases such as cancer. A cure in most chronic diseases is always difficult to achieve, regardless of the treatment modalities used. However, in NICO (neuralgia-inducing cavitational osteonecrosis) patients, when atypical facial pain is present, an 80% cure rate as measured by complete elimination or significant reduction of pain can be expected after the cavitations have been properly debrided.

NICO certainly is a good example of a disease process directly related to a cavitation.

We are continually amazed at the diverse disease states that show marked improvement after the elimination of different sources of dental toxicity. Of course, any treatment success is also significantly supported by proper nutrition, optimal supplementation, stress management, and any of a host of other factors that interrelate to affect our health in both positive and negative ways. However, dental toxicity truly appears to be a significant cause of, or contributor to, many chronic diseases.

What if I don't get better after the extraction of a root canal treated tooth or after cavitation surgery?

This is certainly possible. Not everybody shows dramatic improvements in health and some people may not show any improvement. This means that oral disease is not the predominant cause of a given disease, or that there may be other more significant factors that are contributing to a given disease, or that irreversible damage has already been done. Sometimes improvement may take a long time and require some of the adjunctive therapies mentioned above. For example, if a patient has a systemic yeast infection that initially developed due to immune suppression from the toxicity of a cavitation or a root canal treated tooth, the patient may not get well until the primary focus is removed (the cavitation) *and* the patient is treated for systemic yeast infection. Simply treating the cavitation will only eliminate the primary focus that started the disease and not the secondary infection that has already spread systemically. Once the fire has been started, snuffing out the match that started it will not put out the fire.

Should antibiotics be used during extractions and cavitation surgery?

We feel that antibiotics should be used during surgery. The reason we believe that antibiotics are necessary is because there are over 400 different species of bacteria in the mouth. Many bacteria can be released into the bloodstream during the surgical procedure and may then travel to other sites in the body to begin a secondary infection. By administering antibiotics during surgery, we hope to destroy any bacteria that escape into the bloodstream and thus prevent a new infection in another part of the body.

We also feel that antibiotics are over-prescribed, often improperly used, and usually administered for too long a period of time. The overzealous use of antibiotics has led to antibiotic-resistant strains of bacteria as well as to the disruption of the delicate balance of good bacteria in the body. This can cause other serious problems to develop. For example, antibiotic use can result in yeast infections in areas such as the gastrointestinal tract that can be very difficult to cure. We feel that the risk-to-benefit ratio favors the judicious use of antibiotics during these oral surgery procedures.

Sanum remedies, which actually deliberately introduce live microbes into the area treated, are not effective replacements for antibiotics during and after surgery. There simply is no proof of efficacy, and there is no scientific reason to believe that they should work. Some reports indicate Sanum remedies can impair healing and possibly even increase the size of a cavitation into which they are injected. This is not surprising since any of a number of different live microbes, as are also found in a Sanum remedy injection, can be expected to become toxic when they are trapped in sites significantly deprived of oxygen.

Sizeable doses of vitamin C, both intravenously and orally, are highly effective in eliminating a wide range of infections and in promoting good healing and strong immune function. 50 to 100 grams given intravenously over several hours may sometimes be required to assure the rapid recovery of sicker patients with weaker immune systems. Depending upon bowel tolerance (vitamin C can cause diarrhea) and the health of the kidneys, 5 to 15 grams of oral sodium ascorbate daily in divided doses should also be given to most patients following surgey to support their health and maintain their recoveries. Some patients may require a lesser dose of vitamin C, and a significant number of patients may even require a larger dose. This type of vitamin C dosing must be accompanied by at least two quarts of purified water daily.

How can the risk of infection be reduced during oral surgery?

We already mentioned the use of antibiotics during surgery. The administration of postoperative antibiotics will be case-dependent and must be discussed individually with your surgeon. It is important to have a good tooth cleaning approximately one week before surgery if possible. The proper administration of antibiotics should also accompany such a cleaning of the teeth. In addition, laser curettage of the gums around the teeth will destroy any bacteria present in the gum pockets around the teeth and lessen the subsequent introduction of bacteria into the surgical site.

Laser curettage is a procedure where a low power laser is placed around the teeth and under the gum in the space that surrounds the teeth called the periodontal sulcus. This is the area where most of the bacteria live, and it is the site where periodontal disease usually begins. This treatment is virtually painless when used with a topically applied anesthetic. Laser curettage can be done in the weeks before surgery to reduce the bacteria levels in the gums. It should also be performed by your surgeon immediately prior to surgery.

An antimicrobial mouth rise such as chlorhexidine gluconate 0.12% or Therasol should be used immediately prior to surgery. Your surgeon may also instruct you to use a similar mouth rinse several days prior to surgery as well to further reduce the chances of post-operative infection.

What should I do first: have my amalgams replaced or have my root canal treated teeth extracted and my cavitations cleaned?

Although there are exceptions, we feel that the extraction of root canal treated teeth and the cleaning of cavitations should be addressed first. This allows for the quickest recovery of the immune system possible, since the toxins in root canal treated teeth and cavitations appear to be much more toxic than the mercury-containing amalgam fillings.

Is there any way to tell if my root canal is toxic?

There is a test that may be useful in demonstrating the toxicity of *some* root canal treated teeth in the mouth. This test looks for toxins that are contained in the tiny amounts of fluid that are expressed between the gum and the tooth. However, we cannot conclude that a negative toxicity test result means that the root canal treated tooth is not infected or toxic. It simply means that the toxins are not present in the gum tissue around the crown part of the tooth where the sample is taken from. There most certainly is some degree of infection deep within the bone around the tip of the root, and the toxins may not migrate to the top part of the tooth where the sample is taken for analysis. Also, there are nearly always some circumstances under which a given test is simply not accurate.

If a tooth presents a positive toxicity test then it must be determined whether the toxicity is from a tooth infection, a gum infection, or both. A control tooth in the same mouth must also be analyzed since many of the bacterial toxins can easily travel from one site in the mouth to another site. Therefore, a positive toxicity test on a tooth may be the result of toxicity occurring somewhere else in the mouth that has migrated to the test tooth.

To the best of our knowledge, toxicity testing has always demonstrated significant toxins in an extracted root canal tooth, regardless of the results that were previously obtained on the surrounding crevicular fluid, and very many to date have now been tested. Furthermore, all cavitation samples tested have also demonstrated significant toxicity as measured by the degree of vital enzyme inhibition caused by the cavitation sample.

In summary, we are absolutely convinced that the root canal procedure is fatally flawed, *always* resulting in an infected and toxic tooth, even in the rare event when infection was not present prior to the procedure. We do not feel there are any exceptions to this conclusion. We feel that any root canal treated tooth that is allowed to remain in the mouth will eventually have a negative impact on the patient's health. Furthermore, the root canal treated tooth will always be expected to continually stress and compromise the immune system in ways which may not be clincally apparent from the time the root canal procedure is originally performed.

11

PATIENT TESTIMONIALS

Otherwise Untreatable Headaches

Since an early teen, I have had a few root canals on various teeth in the upper left side of my mouth. In early 1999, I started to develop headaches that began on the left temple and radiated to the back of my head, behind my ear and my eye. The pain would come and go and I dealt with it for as long as I could. I had been seeing my dentist regularly for check-ups and cleanings; in the spring of 1999, I required another root canal in the same spot, the upper left side. During the series of root canal visits, the pain intensified; I was taking four Advil every four hours to alleviate the pain. I could have used something stronger but I could not take narcotics and continue to work as a nurse. The dentist did try to make an accurate diagnosis of my pain but stated that he felt that it was unrelated to my teeth. I proceeded to have a MRI, a visit with an Ear, Nose, and Throat doctor as well as a full exam with a neurologist. All findings were negative and the headaches remained a mystery. I returned to my dentist and not being able to make a definitive diagnosis he suggested we pull the tooth that was last root canal treated. It took four weeks to heal because I developed a dry socket. I now was on narcotics, Vicodin to be exact, and still had no relief from headaches. This pain was the worst I have ever experienced; it felt like I had a hole in my gum that was open to the nerves in my face. Ultimately, the gum healed but the headaches persisted. Again, my dentist recommended a pain clinic to me since he could find nothing dentally wrong.

Understanding now that I was at a dead end, I was speaking to my mother-in-law who told me about Dr. Bob Kulacz. She explained that he was "very bright" and that he practiced "biological dentistry". When I asked her to explain she stated "he takes your whole body into consideration when you have a problem, not just your teeth."

I had nothing to lose; I called Dr. Kulacz in August of 1999. I explained my symptoms to him over the phone; right then and there, he said "it sounds like you have some type of circulation problem to the bone and possible residual infection or dead bone where the extractions were performed. Come and see me right away." I saw Dr. Kulacz the next day. Within minutes, he had made a definitive diagnosis. "Your pain is from the damage that was caused by use of novacaine with vasoconstrictors during all of the root canals you have had. In addition, all root canals you had were infected. I would like to remove the affected teeth and infected, dead bone at the extraction sites and your pain will likely be resolved". I had the surgery a day or two later and my headaches were finally gone. Subsequently, I had a partial bridge placed and have *never* had the same headache return.

Dr. Kulacz through his knowledge and wisdom truly saved me from a life of pain and potential death from the infection that could have spread to my blood stream. In addition, as a health care provider he has proven that you MUST consider the whole body; not just the teeth. Most dentists don't get involved in the medical history of their patients and most physicians don't get involved with the dental history of their patients. I am so grateful that Dr. Kulacz took the time to listen to me, analyze my symptoms, and make the right decisions to alleviate my pain and let me go on with a normal life. He is truly an incredible dentist and human being.

-T.D., R.N., B.S.N., Mahopac, NY

The following is an example of a *typical* pathology report on a sample from the site of a root canal treated tooth or from the site of a cavitation. Although this report specifies the location of the sample as tooth # 15, this sample also includes bone from the extracted root canal tooth #14 that developed a dry socket after extraction. As in medicine, all diseased tissue removed from the body should be subject to biopsy. Many of the pathology reports on patients show similar if not more severe pathological conditions. (This pathology report is from the above patient T.D. of Mahopac, NY)

Head & Neck Diagnostics of America
A Division of The Maxillofacial Center
for Diagnostics & Research
165 Scott Avenue, Suite 101, Morgantown, WV 26508
Phone: 304-292-4429 Fax: 304-291-5649

BIOPSY REPORT #HN99-2588
Surgery date: 8/18/99
Date received: 8/23/99
Date completed: 8/31/99

SURGEON:
Dr. Robert Kulacz
280 Mamaroneck Ave, STE 307

White Plains, NY 10605
914-288-0993
Fax: 914-288-0978

PATIENT:
T.D.
AGE (yrs.)/
GENDER:33FD

SOURCE OF SPECIMEN (location): **UL #15**.
CLINICAL DIAGNOSIS/DESCRIPTION: **Pulpitis.**

GROSS DESCRIPTION OF TISSUE RECEIVED:

PART A: The specimen consists of multiple cancellous, hemorrhagic, hard and partially softened bone fragments measuring 0.7xO.4xO.2 cm in aggregation. The entire specimen is decalcified.
PART B: The specimen consists of a tooth. Sections will be submitted after decalcification.

MICROSCOPIC DESCRIPTION OF TISSUE:
PART A: Sections show globules of a gray/translucent foreign material coated by PMNs and coccal bacterial colonies. PMNs are also seen with lymphocytes in small fragments of necrotic fibrovascular tissue. There is no evidence of malignancy.
PART B: Cross sections through the apical portions of the roots show one with generalized fibrosis and moderate dystrophic calcification, with peripheral edema and considerably dilated apical veins and lymphatics. The other pulps show less fibrosis and more edema and the dilated veins are not as severely enlarged. Attached periodontal ligament fragments are unremarkable. There is no evidence of malignancy.
MICROSCOPIC DIAGNOSIS:
PART A: Consistent with subacute osteomyelitis with foreign material and bacterial colonies, maxillary left first molar area.
PART B: Chronic fibrosing and calcific pulpitis with congestion and peripheral edema (combined acute and chronic pulpitis,) maxillary left second molar.
NOTE: Although we traditionally consider pulpal edema and congestion to be evidence of acute pulpitis, it could also be evidence of a chronic outflow problem. The PART A diagnosis is presumably from area #14, but would also be consistent with a periodontal abscess if #15 had a pocket associated with it. The foreign material in PART A is consistent with endodontic materials.

PATHOLOGIST: J.E. Bouquot, D.D.S, M.S.D., Director

Chronic Arthritis Relief

There is no way I can thank you enough for helping me to get back to an active life again.

As you know I was wearing a brace on my knee, so I could hold off getting a knee replacement. I did get some relief.

Since you extracted two bottom teeth, which were infected, I have not been wearing my knee brace. I'm able to play golf and walk without discomfort. Overall, my arthritis is about 85% better.

Thank you
And
God Bless
-M.D., New York

Facial Neuralgia

Dear Dr. Kulacz:

Today marks the beginning of a new lease on life for me. I had a wonderful day thinking about how lucky I am to finally get a second chance to enjoy all those things with which I am so truly blessed. You know my story; but just for the record, I will summarize.

This past January, I decided to bridge my lower left molars: That was the sorriest day of my life. Each and every aspect of my life was compromised from that point on. I endured the most excruciating pain I had every experienced in my entire life which includes a 20-hour labor and delivery. My mouth was numbed repeatedly during endodontic procedures, many times without success. I experienced temporary face paralysis and repeated infections as well as many, many extremely unpleasant procedures—all without relieving any of my pain. The only way I was able to make it through each day was with the help of my very supportive friends and family. There were many nights I did not want to face another day and began to understand why people end their lives.

Short of pulling two teeth out of my mouth, I was referred to a neurologist who diagnosed me with facial neuralgia and prescribed Neurontin. The pain was somewhat relieved but I was unable to function as I am accustomed due to extreme fatigue and forgetfulness. The pain did eventually return and intensify.

As a last resort, I chose an alternative route—acupuncture. Fortunately for me, my Family Nurse Practitioner and Acupuncturist had just met you and thought you could possibly help me. After my conversation with you, I was upset to hear that the teeth I had been holding onto in vain would have to be removed and the bone tissue cleaned out properly. At that point, I was way beyond the "end of my rope" so I consented to the surgery. All the information I received from you and Dr. Karen Shrimplin was truly remarkable and professional and I had no doubt you would indeed help me.

I wasn't the slightest bit nervous going into the procedure. The procedure itself was painless, without incident. You and your anesthesiologist, Dr. Greenspan, were a pleasure to deal with, and I will be an advocate in your crusade to educate those who suffer needlessly.

-T.S., New Jersey

The following two pathology reports are for T.S. of New Jersey.

Head & Neck Diagnostic of America
A Division of The Maxillofacial Center for Diagnostics & Research
165 Scott Avenue, Suite 101, Morgantown, WV 26508
Phone: 304-292-4429 Fax: 304-291-5649

BIOPSY REPORT #HN99-3872
Surgery date: 11/18/99
Date received: 11/24/99
Date completed: 12/1/99

SURGEON:
Dr. Robert Kulacz

PATIENT:
T.S.

280 Mamaroneck Avenue, Great Meadows, NJ
Suite 307 White Plains, NY Age/ Gender: 44F
10605 Date of Birth: 1/29/55
914-288-0993 fax 914-288-0978

SOURCE OF SPECIMEN (location): Lower left
CLINICAL DIAGNOSIS/DESCRIPTION: NICO

GROSS DESCRIPTION OF TISSUE RECEIVED:
The specimen consists of multiple irregular and partially hemorrhagic calcified tissue fragments measuring 0.4x0.4x0.3 cm in aggregation. These are decalcified as PART A. Also included is mandibular molar and bicuspid with endodontic therapy and removed crowns. These are decalcified as PART B.

MICROSCOPIC DESCRIPTION OF TISSUE:
PART A: Sections show cortical bone with mild osteoblastic activity and occasional microcracking, with only occasional missing osteocytes. There are excess cement lines, as there are in underlying thicker than normal but sparsely spaced bony trabeculae. Trabeculae also show occasional missing osteocytes. Available fatty marrow shows a generalized wispy reticular fatty degeneration with small numbers of chronic inflammatory cells and scattered mast cells. Marrow veins are dilated and one area shows a pale staining granular fat necrosis with sprinkled erythrocytes, consistent with microinfarction. There is no evidence of malignancy.

PART B: Cross sections through the apical portions of the roots show two apical canals with abundant necrotic pulpal debris adjacent to endodontic materials with one also showing moderately severe internal resorption. Attached periodontal ligament is unremarkable. There is no evidence of malignancy.

MICROSCOPIC DIAGNOSIS:

PART A: Bone marrow edema with scattered chronic inflammatory cells (variant of ischemic osteonecrosis), left mandibular second molar and first bicuspid areas.

PART B: Necrotic pulpal remnants in apical canals of endodontically treated tooth, mandibular left second molar and first bicuspid.

NOTE: Most of the necrotic debris and internal root resorption is in the molar.

PATHOLOGIST: J.E. Bouquot, D.D.S., M.S.D., Director

Head & Neck Diagnostic of America
A Division of The Maxillofacial Center for Diagnostics & Research
165 Scott Avenue, Suite 101, Morgantown, WV 26508
Phone: 304-292-4429 Fax: 304-291-5649

BIOPSY REPORT #HN99-3934
Surgery date: 11/18/99
Date received: 12/1/99
Date completed: 12/7/99

SURGEON:
Dr. Robert Kulacz
280 Mamaroneck Avenue,
Suite 307 White Plains, NY
10605
914-288-0993 fax 914-288-0978

PATIENT:
T.S.
Great Meadows, NJ
Age/ Gender: 44F
Date of Birth: 1/29/55

SOURCE OF SPECIMEN(location): #30
CLINICAL DIAGNOSIS/ DESCRIPTION: 1) Periapical granuloma 2) Osteonecrosis

GROSS DESCRIPTION OF TISSUE RECEIVED:
The specimen consists of three of very small and nonhemorrhagic calcified tissue fragments measuring 0.3x0.2x0.1 cm in aggregation. This portion is decalcified as PART A. Also included are two fractured molar roots which have been endodontically treated and have a yellow color and these are decalcified as PART B.

MICROSCOPIC DESCRIPTION OF TISSUE:
PART A: Sections show viable cortical bone with prominent osteoid rimming and occasional osteoblastic activity. The bone appears viable but underlying bony trabeculae are thicker than normal and show excess cement lines with scattered missing osteocytes. A fragment of moderately dense collagenic connective tissue shows a degenerated stratified squamous lining epithelium along edges and contains moderate numbers of chronic inflammatory cells. Available marrow spaces are filled with a very loose fibrosis connective tissue with dilated veins and capillaries. There is no evidence of malignancy.

PART B: Cross sections through the apical portions of the roots show abundant necrotic pulpal debris and hemorrhage in all apical canals, admixed with endodontic materials and sometimes with chronic inflammatory cells. One apical canal has only a small amount of endodontic material within it. There is no evidence of malignancy.

MICROSCOPIC DIAGNOSIS:
PART A: Chronically inflamed periapical cyst with chronic sclerosing osteomyelitis (condensing ostetitis) of surrounding bone, mandibular right first molar area.

PART B: Nonsuppurative pulpal necrosis of endodontically treated tooth, mandibular right first molar.

NOTE: The osteosclerosis here may not have been prominent enough to be obvious radiographically.

PATHOLOGIST: J.E. Bouquot, D.D.S., M.S.D., Director

Largely Pain-Free

Dr. Kulacz performed cavitational surgery in the sites of three of my extracted wisdom teeth on July 12, 2000.

I was referred to Dr. Kulacz by my local dentist in Pennsylvania, because an ultrasound test indicated that I had fairly deep cavitations in my lower jaw on both right and left sides. In addition, one of my friends had recently undergone extensive cavitational surgery by Dr. Kulacz and highly recommended him to me.

Before undergoing surgery, I was given a packet of information including forms to be completed concerning my health history, information about techniques that would be used in my surgery, and pre-and post-surgical protocol. I was glad both to be well informed myself and that Dr. Kulacz would be well informed about my condition before my surgery. This information also assured me that much care would be taken to safeguard my health and to prevent further infection.

On the day of my surgery, my husband and I were given more than adequate time to discuss matters with Dr. Kulacz. Having heard various stories and rumors, I was somewhat concerned about possible nerve damage. Dr. Kulacz, by showing me photos of someone else's surgery, explained that the larger nerves were encased in something like a sheaf, and that there was essentially no reason to fear that they would be injured.

We also discussed the area of my previously extracted upper right wisdom tooth. Although the cavitat test had shown no problem in that area, Dr. Kulacz said that my panorex x-ray seemed to suggest that there might be a cavitation in that area as well. As he was concerned, he offered to check out that area also at no extra cost to me, and we agreed that this was the wise thing to do.

The general anesthesia was performed by an anesthesiologist whom Dr. Kulacz highly trusts and respects. The experience of the surgery during anesthesia was somewhat like a pleasant dream. After the IV was inserted, I began to feel sleepy, and before I knew it, I was barely conscious of anything except perhaps a vague sound of drilling. Then the next thing I knew, the surgery, which had really lasted about 3 hours, was over.

Dr. Kulacz seemed quite happy about the surgery even though he had found quite large cavitations; he had been able to successfully remove much of the infection in my jaw. He had found a large cavitation even in the upper right jaw, the area that had shown only a suggestion of a problem on the x-ray. We were so glad that we had decided to check out that area in addition to the more obvious ones.

Healing from the surgery took place quickly and easily. I fully expected to need painkillers after the anesthesia lost its effect, but the pain was so minimal that I didn't need any. Thirteen days after the surgery I went to my local dentist to have the sutures removed. He and his assistant both seemed surprised that I had healed so well already. I also went to a clinic in Switzerland the following month and the doctor there also exclaimed, "Good job!" when he looked in my mouth.

-C.H., Pennsylvania

Congestive Heart Failure

The following patient had a heart attack at age 40, a second heart attack nine years later that was treated with coronary bypass surgery, and at age 62 is currently in congestive heart failure and awaiting a heart transplant. He presented with severe periodontal disease as well as acute endodontic infections.

Head & Neck Diagnostic of America
A Division of The Maxillofacial Center for
Diagnostics & Research
165 Scott Avenue, Suite 101, Morgantown, WV 26508
Phone: 304-292-4429 Fax: 304-291-5649

BIOPSY REPORT #HN2001-4717
Surgery date: 11/14/01
Date received: 11/28/01
Date completed: 12/4/01

SURGEON:
Dr. Robert Kulacz
280 Mamaroneck Avenue,
Suite 307 White Plains, NY
10605
914-288-0993 fax 914-288-0978

PATIENT:
L.M.
Armonk, NY
Age/ Gender: 61M
Date of Birth: 3/13/40

SOURCE OF SPECIMEN (location): 31,32
CLINICAL DIAGNOSIS/DESCRIPTION: 1)granuloma 2)osteonecrosis, osteomyelitis

GROSS DESCRIPTION OF TISSUE RECEIVED:
The specimen consists of multiple irregular and tan soft and hard tissue fragments measuring 0.4x0.4x0.3 cm in aggregation. These are decalcified as Part A. Also included is a mandibular molar with a golden crown, and two fractured and separate roots, all decalcified as Part B.

MICROSCOPIC DESCRIPTION OF TISSUE:
Part A: Sections show fragments of dense collagenic connective tissue with focal infiltration by moderate numbers of chronic inflammatory cells and occasional PMNs. Focal necrosis is seen and bone from the apparent lesional periphery shows surface osteoblastic activity and only occasional missing osteocytes.

Immature or newly forming bone is seen but has lymphocytes in its stroma, and the stroma is sometimes degenerated. Mixed bacterial colonies are seen but are unattached, hence, are presumed to be surface artifact. Marrow vessels are sometimes greatly dilated. A small amount fatty marrow is seen and shows ischemic myleofibrosis with infiltration by occasional lymphocytes. There is no evidence of malignancy.

Part B: Cross sections through the tooth show viable apical pulp tissue except in one root which has necrotic pulpal debris in a canal, along with numerous PMNs. The latter canal has multiple sites of inner dentin wall destruction and there is no evidence of malignancy.

MICROSCOPIC DIAGNOSIS:
Part A: Subacutely inflamed periapical granuloma, and chronic nonsuppurative osteomyelitis of newly forming bone (chronically inflamed new bone), and with ischemic marrow damage, mandibular right second and third molar area.

Part B: Suppurative pulpal necrosis, with internal root resorption, mandibular right second or third molar.

PATHOLOGIST: J.E. Bouquot, D.D.S., M.S.D., Director

Headache and Sinus Congestion

The following patient presented with a constant headache for one year duration as well as chronic sinus congestion in the left sinus. Both his dentist and an ear, nose, and throat specialist found no pathology or cause for his condition. After removing tooth #14 which was treated with a root canal, both his headaches and sinus congestion were immediately alleviated.

Head & Neck Diagnostic of America

A Division of The Maxillofacial Center for Diagnostics & Research
165 Scott Avenue, Suite 101, Morgantown, WV 26508
Phone: 304-292-4429 Fax: 304-291-5649

BIOPSY REPORT #HN2000-1279
Surgery date: 4/4/00
Date received: 4/7/00
Date completed: 4/17/00

SURGEON:
Dr. Robert Kulacz
280 Mamaroneck Avenue,
Suite 307 White Plains,
10605
914-288-0993 fax 914-288-0978

PATIENT:
C.C.
Ridgefield. CT
NY Age/ Gender: 60M
Date of Birth: 3/20/40

SOURCE OF SPECIMEN(location): #14
CLINICAL DIAGNOSIS/ DESCRIPTION: Osteonecrosis/ osteomyelitis.

GROSS DESCRIPTION OF TISSUE RECEIVED: The specimen consists of multiple irregular and dirty tan calcified tissue fragments measuring 0.7x0.4x0.2 cm in aggregation. These are decalcified as PART A. Also included are three endodontically treated root tips, two with periapical soft tissue attached, and these are decalcified as PART B.

MICROSCOPIC DESCRIPTION OF TISSUE:
PART A: Sections show thick cortical and trabecular bone with occasional osteoblastic activity and with only occasional missing osteocytes. Marrow spaces show areas of reticular fatty degeneration with dilated capillaries, and some areas show a moderately dense and focally edematous fibrosis with scat-

tered chronic inflammatory cells in moderate numbers. There is no evidence of malignancy.

PART B: Cross sections through the apical portions of the roots show abundant necrotic debris adjacent to endodontic materials in two apical canals, with chronic inflammatory cells in one canal. There is no evidence of malignancy.

MICROSCOPIC DIAGNOSIS:
PART A: Periapical granuloma with chronic nonsuppurative osteomyelitis of surrounding bone, maxillary left first molar area.

PART B: Nonsuppurative pulpal necrosis of endodontically treated tooth, maxillary left first molar.

PATHOLOGIST: J.E. Bouquot, D.D.S., M.S.D., Director

Heart Attack

The following patient had a recent heart attack. He presented with several severe dental infections.

Head & Neck Diagnostic of America
A Division of The Maxillofacial Center for Diagnostics & Research
165 Scott Avenue, Suite 101, Morgantown, WV 26508
Phone: 304-292-4429 Fax: 304-291-5649

BIOPSY REPORT #HN2001-4892
Surgery date: 4/4/00
Date received: 4/7/00
Date completed: 4/17/00

SURGEON: PATIENT:
Dr. Robert Kulacz R.S.
280 Mamaroneck Avenue, Mahopac, NY
Suite 307 White Plains, NY Age/ Gender: 63M
10605 Date of Birth: 7/7/38
914-288-0993 fax 914-288-0978

SOURCE OF SPECIMEN(location): #15
CLINICAL DIAGNOSIS/ DESCRIPTION: Osteomyelitis.

GROSS DESCRIPTION OF TISSUE RECEIVED:
The specimen consists of multiple irregular and dirty tan and focal hemorrhagic soft and hard tissue fragments measuring 0.6x0.5x0.4 cm in aggregation. These are decalcified as Part A. Also included is a maxillary molar with removed crown and dilacerated roots and this is decalcified as Part B.

MICROSCOPIC DESCRIPTION OF TISSUE:
PART A: Sections show a fragment of degenerated fibrous connective tissue with infiltration by a large number of chronic inflammatory cells. One edge has a degenerated stratified squamous lining epithelium along it, with PMNs seen within and beneath this epithelium. Fragments of bone from the apparent lesional periphery show occasional missing osteocytes and show marrow spaces filled with loose fibrous tissue with myxoid degeneration and occasional scattered lymphocytes. A separate mixed bacterial colony is presumed to be surface artifact, and there is no evidence of malignancy.

PART B: Cross sections through the tooth show complete replacement of apical canal contents by endodontic materials in two apical canals, with necrotic pulpal remnants admixed with endodontic materials in one apical canal. Inflammatory cells are not seen in the canal but are numerous within the attached granulation tissue. There is no evidence of malignancy

MICROSCOPIC DIAGNOSIS:
PART A: Subacutely inflamed periapical cyst, with mild chronic nonsuppurative osteomyelitis of surrounding bone, maxillary left second molar area.

PART B: Necrotic pulpal remnants in apical canal of endodontically treated tooth, maxillary left second molar.

PATHOLOGIST: J.E. Bouquot, D.D.S., M.S.D., Director

Hearing Loss and Sinus Infection
G.R.B
Rahway, NJ

Dr. George Meinig
C/O Bion Publishing
P.O. BOX 10
Ojal, CA 93024

January 28, 2002

Dear Dr. Meinig:

I just wanted to take the time to thank you first of all for writing such an informative book, *Root Canal Cover-up*. It really made me even more aware of the possible connection between my poor health and my root canals. Even though the sad journey started for me over 10 years ago when I had my first root canal, I am thankful that the worst is over. I am now root canal free. I had a total of three removed all were infected.

I was suffering from severe stomach problems that started months after my first root canal. I was even hospitalized for Pancreatitis. The 7-day hospital stay cost over $25,000 and none of the specialists could find out what was causing the symptoms. They gave me medicine to relieve the symptoms but never could get to the root of the cause.

As you can see as you read my health history, it took several more years but finally I did find relief. I hope my body can full recover from the years of infection and leeching metals. Right now I feel better than I have in years.

And that brings me to my final reason for this letter. I really want to thank you for referring me to Dr. Robert Kulacz. He was brave and skilled enough to venture into my sinus cavity and clean out the infection. He told me on the day of the surgery that if the infection returned that it was because there was a secondary infection in my upper sinus area that he could not reach. He said the ENT Doctor would easily be able to help me with any residual infection. But that was not necessary, Dr. Kulacz cleaned the area so thoroughly that he must have gotten all the infection because it has not returned. So thanks again for the referral, for your book, and for having the integrity to tell the truth.

-G.R.B.

CC: Dr. Robert Kulacz

G.R.B.-Health History

Jan-91	1st root canal performed (lower right molar)
Dec-91	Stomach problems begin. Scattered episodes of stomach pain at night that would radiate to back area.
Mar-92	Pain diagnosed as pancreatitis. Hospitalized for one week. Cause: "unknown."
Mar-97	Symptoms return, unable to eat. Endoscopy and ultrasound performed. Cause of symptoms: "unknown"
Mar-98	2nd root canal performed (lower left molar)

Apr-99	3rd (last) root canal performed (upper left molar) Few weeks after procedure, I noticed cap did not fit properly. While flossing I could feel a gap in back of cap.
Dec-99	Health worsens. Chronically fatigued, could not do household chores without rest. Stomach symptoms worse than ever. (nausea, terrible gas, heartburn.) Also, night sweats and numbing of fingers. Noticed that hearing in left ear is diminished.
Feb-00	Decided to try change of diet, symptoms still persist.
Apr-00	Reluctant to return to Gastrointestinal Specialist, I decided to give alternative medicine a try. Homeopathic Practitioner found my body to be filled with parasites, bacteria, viruses, and metals.
Jan-01	Homeopathy temporarily helped but bacteria in my stomach kept returning. I began to suspect that the bacteria were somehow coming from within my body. Read books by Dr. Clark and Dr. Meinig and became aware of the root canal connection.

Discussed issue with my dentist (who performed the last 2 root canals):

1. He admitted that the horrible stench in my mouth (I smelled it when he inserted rubber dam) was due to bacteria from my root canals.
2. Yet, he refused to believe that the same bacteria was causing my stomach problems. Therefore, he refused to remove root canalled teeth. Referred me to a root canal specialist.
3. Specialist said root canals looked good on X-ray. *But could not say for certain that bacteria was not causing*

my problem. Requested to be informed if once root canals were removed my symptoms improved.

Feb-01	Found a dentist willing to extract my root canals. 1st tooth (lower right molar) took almost 2 hours to remove. Dentist said while bone immediately around tooth was extremely dense the inner bone was soft, infected, and mushy.
Mar-01	Some relief, but stomach still very sensitive. Tired and nauseous all the time. Cap on upper molar falls off while flossing. The inside of cap completely blackened and filled with food particles, horrible smell. Felt immediate relief to my stomach once cap was gone. Now convinced that this tooth was a big problem and had to be removed.
Apr-01	Upper molar extracted. Very difficult extraction, arrived 2pm for appointment, extraction took some 3 hours. Left office at 5:15pm completely traumatized. Dentist said tooth was completely infected; it cracked as it was being pulled and a horrible stench filled the room. Dentist informed my sinus was perforated.
	Even though the extraction was traumatic, almost immediately after extraction stomach symptoms, fatigue, and nausea were gone and have not returned. Once week later, I had a new problem, my sinus became badly infected (area where tooth was). Green mucus coming from nose. Dentist prescribes amoxicillin for sinus. Sinus infection persists. Left earache off and on.

Aug-01	Return to dentist. Sinus still infected. More amoxicillin prescribed, directed to use sinus irrigator. 3rd root canal removed (lower left molar). Dentist found "wicked infection," an performed cavitation surgery.
Dec-01	My father dies, immunity lowered. Sinus infection goes crazy with green mucous pouring out of left nostril and left eye socket painful and swollen. Left ear aches constantly. Made appointment with Ear, Nose, and Throat Specialist. Doctor agrees I have a sinus infection and confirms that I have hearing loss in my left ear. Prescribes 3 weeks of antibiotics (Cefin). Three weeks later-infection persists… Returning to dentist begging him to clean out area where upper left molar was extracted and clean sinus. Dentist refuses says he sees nothing on x-ray. Says socket is healing well. He does not believe the sinus condition is related to extracted tooth.
Jan-02	Called Dr. George Meinig in California. Referred to Dr. Robert Kulacz, NY. Dr. Kulacz performed oral surgery and after extracting a dead upper left molar, he cleaned out the site of the original root canal and courageously entered sinus area to clean. Found horrible cyst in sinus cavity. Drained and cleaned out cyst and surrounding dead bone and tissue.

One Week After Surgery:

A Miracle! The sinus infection is gone. No traces of it, and I feel wonderful. I am finally symptom free, with no root canals in my mouth,

Still partially deaf in left ear, I believe this will always serve as a reminder to me of just how dangerous to one's health root canals can be.

APPENDIX I

SURGICAL PROTOCOL FOR TOOTH EXTRACTIONS AND CAVITATION SURGERY

General Observations

Tooth extractions and cavitation debridement are surgical procedures performed in the oral cavity that involve both the soft tissues of the mouth, such as the gingiva, and the bones of the maxilla and mandible. Strict adherence to surgical protocols, such as those practiced by orthopedic surgeons, should also apply to oral surgery procedures. Unfortunately, dentistry has been slow to adopt the surgical principles practiced in medicine that are vital to successful surgical outcome. We must remember that dentists, as surgeons of the oral cavity, are still operating on bone. Although the mouth is a more forgiving place to operate in terms of the healing of soft tissue, infected bone is difficult to completely heal no matter where in the body it is located. In fact, bone infection in the mouth is probably *more* likely to become chronic and entrenched than bone infection elsewhere in the body. Furthermore, the ability of the mouth to rapidly heal soft tissue infections tends to make many dentists feel that infected bone in the mouth will heal just as readily, which is definitely not the case. We now know how easily cavitations develop, and the seemingly complete healing after many routine dental extractions is clearly an illusion. Accepted surgical procedures must be followed everywhere in the body in order to optimize the chances of complete healing and complete clinical recovery.

Protocol

1. A complete patient medical and dental history, including consultation with all treating physicians, is essential *before* treatment is rendered. As the mouth is not isolated from the rest of the body, such a complete history is important. Nearly all dental procedures, especially surgery, have systemic, body-wide implications.
2. A thorough dental evaluation of the hard and soft tissues of the oral cavity is essential. The examination should include all necessary x-rays, along with a complete clinical exam that includes pulp vitality tests of the teeth to determine which teeth are healthy and alive and which teeth might be unexpectedly nerve-dead and nonvital. Any additional tests that may aid in diagnosis and treatment planning should also be performed. It is important to point out that pulp vitality tests are an *integral part* in assessing the health of the teeth that did not receive root canal treatments. Reliance solely on modalities such as electrodermal screening and Cavitat screening in place of electric pulp testing to diagnose and determine tooth vitality is, in our opinion, misguided and inappropriate. Leaving a dead, nonvital tooth behind can be as serious as leaving behind a root canal treated tooth. Root canal treated teeth do not need the

pulp vitality testing since they uniformly fail it, as would be logically expected.
3. After the initial assessment of the patient's condition, a treatment plan must be established. If the treatment plan includes extractions and/or cavitation surgery, it is important to seek a surgeon who is not only surgically skilled, but who also has the ability to deliver intravenous medicines. Intravenous sedation is often necessary, and there must also be an access for the administration of appropriate antibiotics and infection-fighting nutrients such as vitamin C.
4. Alternative treatments such as the injection of various alternative remedies into the site of infection such as the bone around a root canal treated tooth or around other infected teeth should *not* be done. Similarly, no injections should be made into cavitation sites. Many of these treatments actually make the disease process worse. Furthermore, there are some dentists advocating the use of these medicaments *instead* of surgery. It is impossible to restore dead bone to live bone again with any medication. Surgery must be performed to remove all of the dead and infected bone as well as establishing adequate perfusion of blood from adjacent healthy bone into the surgical site. This is the only way healing can occur.
5. Teeth should be cleaned up about two weeks prior to surgery to reduce the amount of bacteria present in the mouth and lessen the chances of post-operative infection. Laser curettage in the sulcus around each tooth can dramatically reduce the presence of bacteria even further.
6. General medical clearance, when appropriate, should be obtained for the day of oral surgery.
7. A written informed consent signed by the patient should be obtained prior to the planned procedure. All poten-

tial complications of the procedure should be thoroughly discussed. It is preferable that a family member also participates in this consent, especially to help verify that all that has been discussed is fully understood. Consideration might be given to a videotaping of the discussion of the consent, which gives the dentist further evidence that all information was discussed and was completely understood by the patient prior to signing the consent form.
8. Preoperative medications such as antibiotics should be administered.
9. The oral cavity should be cleansed with an appropriate antimicrobial agent.
10. Local anesthetic *without* a vasoconstrictor should be used. Vasoconstrictors prevent blood from flowing into the area. Good blood flow to the surgical site is necessary to help assure the best chances of complete healing. Even the transient vasoconstriction produced by anesthetics with a vasoconstrictor can severely compromise the procedure. In addition, the preservatives used in anesthetics containing vasoconstrictors can have negative local as well as systemic effects.
11. If extractions are to take place, the sulcus area around the teeth to be extracted should be treated with a laser to kill the bacteria at the surgical incision site.
12. Surgery should be performed so that the total lesion can be removed. The surgeon must be skilled in operating around the inferior alveolar nerve (the main nerve that runs through the lower jaw) as well as operating through the sinus floor and into the sinus. Many times the lesions seen in cavitations and root canal treated teeth are more extensive than they appear on x-ray. It is important to remove *all* of the diseased tissue. This means that the surgeon should be skilled in operating

around all these anatomical structures. Otherwise, the patient should be referred to another surgeon.
13. Usually, the extraction of an infected or root canal treated tooth requires adequate exposure of the bone surrounding the tooth both for visualization and access to the infected areas. This is obtained by laying a "flap," which simply means that the gum tissue is gently lifted off the bone. I emphasize the word "gently" here since there is a thin layer of tissue that lays directly adjacent to the bone called the periosteum that must be treated with care. The periosteum is the tissue that supplies the outside of the bone with nutrients, and it is also where many of the sensory fibers that can cause post-operative pain are located. It must be treated with respect and handled gently. The kinder you treat the tissue during any operation the less postoperative complications will occur.
14. Surgical sites should be irrigated with saline solution or antibiotic solutions that are acceptable for use in orthopedic surgery. We again must remember that we are operating on bone. Plain water should *never* be used and medications that have not been evaluated for use in bone elsewhere in the body should also never be used for surgical sites in the jawbone.
15. Extractions should be performed as atraumatically as possible. That means that teeth with more than one root such as molars should usually be sectioned and each root removed individually. This technique avoids fractures of the bone and is kinder to the tissues. Dentists were taught in dental school to "expand the socket" by rocking teeth back and force. The term should be "crack the socket" because cortical bone does not stretch and any expansion is obtained by breaking the bone. This should be avoided. Surgical removal of bone when indicated is a much better option and should only be per-

formed with a surgical handpiece (NEVER a dental drill), accompanied by copious sterile saline irrigation (NEVER plain water). Dental drills can introduce air into the surgical site that can form an air embolism. An air embolism is a dangerous situation that can cause death. In addition, dental drills use plain water as an irrigant. This water is not sterile and is not physiologic in terms of salinity. Plain water can cause bone cells to die.

16. Removal of the infected and ischemic bone can be performed initially with a surgical drill at low revolutions per minute with copious irrigation. It is important to keep the temperature of the bone as cool as possible. Aggressive use of a surgical drill will cause an increase in bone temperature due to friction. The bone cells in contact with the drill will die. Dead bone cells are exactly what we are trying to remove and therefore the formation of more dead bone cells must be carefully avoided. Most of the surgical debridement should be performed by hand with surgical curettes.
17. The surgical site must be continuously flushed with an irrigation solution such as 0.9% saline solution.
18. Sometimes bone grafting or sinus closure must be performed. Be sure to discuss this with your surgeon.
19. Closure of the surgical site should be accomplished with sutures.
20. Antibiotics should be given postoperatively to prevent re-infection or systemic dissemination of infection. Intravenous vitamin C is also very important in preventing infection and promoting healing.
21. Strong unipolar magnets over the operative sites greatly accelerate good, complete healing. They also greatly and quickly decrease inflammation and pain at the operative site. The proper side of the magnet must be ap-

plied over the outside of the cheek. The *wrong* side of the magnet can *impair* good healing.
22. Sutures should be removed in seven to ten days.
23. Patients should be instructed to keep pressure on the surgical site by gently biting on surgical gauze. This helps control bleeding as well as keeps the flap close to the bone during the initial healing phase.
24. Ice should be applied to the side of the face for twenty minutes, then removed for twenty minutes. This should be repeated throughout the entire day of surgery but should not be used the following days.
25. The day after surgery the patient should rise with a mild, warm salt water solution (1/4 teaspoon of salt in an 8 oz. glass of water). Do this three to four times per day.

This is a brief outline of surgical principles that should be employed. For a more detailed description of surgical technique look for the upcoming book, tentatively titled *Oral Infections: Diagnosis And Treatment* by Christopher Hussar, D.O., D.D.S., and Robert Kulacz, D.D.S.

APPENDIX II

SELECTED ABSTRACTS FROM THE SCIENTIFIC LITERATURE

All of the following selected abstracts can be readily located online at www.ncbi.nlm.nih.gov/PubMed, which is the website of the National Library of Medicine. Through the search engine service of the National Library of Medicine known as PubMed, many different article abstracts can be readily obtained. Certain articles are available directly in their full text form, while others may be obtained through the Loansome Doc Ordering System or from the direct links to the websites of the publishing journals.

As of the writing of this book, more than 1,650 literature references can be obtained from a PubMed search, typing in: ["focal infection" and dental]. The connection of dental infections and infections throughout the body has very strong literature support. Furthermore, many of these articles are very recent, negating the criticism that focal infection is just an "old" concept.

I. ARTICLES DOCUMENTING THE ASSOCIATIONS BETWEEN DENTAL MICROBES AND SYSTEMIC DISEASE

Article Title:
Dental plaque, platelets, and cardiovascular diseases.

Herzberg MC, Weyer MW.

School of Dentistry, University of Minnesota, Minneapolis, USA.

ABSTRACT: Cardiovascular diseases, including atherosclerosis and myocardial ischemia, occur as a result of a complex set of genetic and environmental factors. During periodontitis, dental plaque microorganisms may disseminate through the blood to infect the vascular endothelium and contribute to the occurrence of atherosclerosis and risk of myocardial ischemia and infarction. Myocardial ischemia and infarction are often preceded by acute thromboembolic events. In an *in vitro* model of thrombosis, certain dental plaque bacteria induce platelets to aggregate. Aggregation of platelets is induced by the platelet aggregation-associated protein [PAAP] expressed on plaque bacteria, including *Streptococcus sanguis* and *Porphyromonas gingivalis*. Intravenous infusion of *S. sanguis* into rabbits has been shown previously to cause changes in the electrocardiogram (ECG), heart rate, blood pressure, and cardiac contractility. These changes are consistent with the occurrence of myocardial infarction. The ECG changes are now shown to begin within 30 seconds after infusion of PAAP+ *S. sanguis*, followed by alterations in blood pressure and respiratory rate. These changes occurred intermittently over a 30-minute period and changed within one heartbeat to a normal pattern and suddenly back to abnormal. Intermittent ECG abnormalities were seen in 13 of 15 rabbits, including left axis deviation, ST-segment depression, preventricular contractions, alternans, and bigemnia. Dose-dependent thrombocytopenia, accumulation of 111Indium-labeled platelets in the lungs, and tachypnea also occurred. No changes occurred with the PAAP-strain. The data indicated that PAPP+ *S. san*guis interacts with circulating platelets, inducing thromboemboli to cause the pulmonary and cardiac abnormalities. During periodontitis, therefore, PAAP+ *S. sanguis* and *P. gingivalis* bacteremia may contribute to the chance of acute thromboembolic events.

From: *Annals of Periodontology* 1998 July; Volume 3, Number 1, pp. 151-160.

Article Title:
Cardiovascular infections: bacterial endocarditis of oral origin. Pathogenesis and prophylaxis.

Nord CE, Heimdahl A.

Department of Microbiology, Huddinge University Hospital, Karolinska Institute, Stockholm, Sweden.

ABSTRACT: The diagnosis infective endocarditis describes infection of the endocardial surface of the heart and indicates the presence of microorganisms in the lesion. In most cases, the heart valves are affected, but the disease can also occur on septal defects or on the mural endocardium. The disease has been classified as acute or subacute based on the progression of the untreated disease. The acute form has a fulminant course with high fever and leukocytosis with death in less than 6 weeks. It is most often associated with infections caused by *Staphylococcus aureus, Streptococcus pneumoniae* or *Streptococcus pyogenes*. The subacute (death within 6 weeks to 3 months) and chronic (death more than 3 months) forms are mostly described together. These forms usually occur in patients with prior valvular disease and are characterized by a slow, indolent course with low-grade fever, night sweats, and weight loss. This form is usually caused by the viridans streptococci. The above-mentioned classification does not include the nonbacterial forms of endocarditis and enterococci often give rise to a disease intermediate between acute and subacute endocarditis. It is preferable to have a classification based on the microorganism responsible since this classification has implications for the course followed and the appropriate antimicrobial agent to use. The clinical manifestations of the disease are so varied that they may be encountered in most medical subspecialties. Successful management is also dependent on the close cooperation of medical and dental disciplines.

From: *Journal of Clinical Periodontology* 1990 August; Volume 17, Number 7 Part 2, pp. 494-496.

Article Title:
Toxic shock syndrome secondary to a dental abscess.

Fardy CH, Findlay G, Owen G, Shortland G.

Department of Child Health, University of Wales College of Medicine, Cardiff.

ABSTRACT: A 9-year-old girl presented with arthralgia and myalgia, which progressed to developing renal failure and overwhelming septic shock. The underlying cause was assumed to be a periodontal abscess from an upper right deciduous canine tooth. The pus from the abscess grew a toxic shock syndrome toxin 1-producing *Staphylococcus aureus*. This case illustrates the importance of an oral surgical review of patients presenting with features of toxic shock syndrome if the source of the infection is not immediately obvious.

From: *International Journal of Oral and Maxillofacial Surgery* 1999 February; Volume 28, Number 1, pp. 60-61.

Article Title:
Identification of periodontal pathogens in atheromatous plaques.

Haraszthy VI, Zambon JJ, Trevisan M, Zeid M, Genco RJ.

Department of Oral Biology, School of Dental Medicine, State University of New York at Buffalo, USA.

ABSTRACT: Recent studies suggest that chronic infections including those associated with periodontitis increase the risk for coronary vascular disease (CVD) and stroke. We hypothesize that oral microorganisms including periodontal bacterial pathogens enter the blood stream during transient bacteremias where they may play a role in the development and progression of atherosclerosis leading to CVD. METHODS: To test this hypothesis, 50 human specimens obtained during carotid endarterectomy were examined for the presence of *Chlamydia pneumoniae*, human cytomegalovirus, and bacterial 16S ribosomal RNA using specific oligonucleotide primers in polymerase chain reaction (PCR) assays. Approximately 100 ng of chromosomal DNA was extracted from each specimen and then amplified using standard conditions (30 cycles of 30 seconds at 95 degrees C, 30 seconds at 55 degrees C, and 30 seconds at

72 degrees C). Bacterial 16S rDNA was amplified using 2 synthetic oligonucleotide primers specific for eubacteria. The PCR product generated with the eubacterial primers was transferred to a charged nylon membrane and probed with digoxigenin-labeled synthetic oligonucleotides specific for *Actinobacillus actinomycetemcomitans*, *Bacteroides forsythus*, *Porphyromonas gingivalis*, and *Prevotella intermedia*. RESULTS: Eighty percent of the 50 endarterectomy specimens were positive in 1 or more of the PCR assays. Thirty-eight percent were positive for HCMV and 18% percent were positive for *C. pneumoniae*. PCR assays for bacterial 16S rDNA also indicated the presence of bacteria in 72% of the surgical specimens. Subsequent hybridization of the bacterial 16S rDNA positive specimens with species-specific oligonucleotide probes revealed that 44% of the 50 atheromas were positive for at least one of the target periodontal pathogens. Thirty percent of the surgical specimens were positive for *B. forsythus*, 26% were positive for *P. gingivalis*, 18% were positive for *A. actinomycetemcomitans*, and 14% were positive for *P. intermedia*. In the surgical specimens positive for periodontal pathogens, more than 1 species was most often detected. Thirteen (59%) of the 22 periodontal pathogen-positive surgical specimens were positive for 2 or more of the target species. CONCLUSIONS: Periodontal pathogens are present in atherosclerotic plaques where, like other infectious microorganisms such as *C. pneumoniae*, they may play a role in the development and progression of atherosclerosis leading to coronary vascular disease and other clinical sequelae.

From: *Journal of Periodontology* 2000 October; Volume 71, Number 10, pp. 1554-1560.

Article Title:
Effects of oral flora on platelets: possible consequences in cardiovascular disease.

Herzberg MC, Meyer MW.

Department of Preventive Sciences, School of Dentistry, University of Minnesota, Minneapolis, USA.

ABSTRACT: During episodes of dental bacteremia, viridans group streptococci encounter platelets. Among these microorganisms, certain *Streptococcus sanguis* induce human and rabbit platelets to aggregate *in vitro*. In experimental rabbits, circulating streptococci induced platelets to aggregate, triggering the accumulation of platelets and fibrin into the heart valve vegetations of endocarditis. At necropsy, affected rabbit hearts showed ischemic areas. We therefore hypothesized that circulating *S. sanguis* might cause coronary thrombosis and signs of myocardial infarction (MI). Signs of MI were monitored in rabbits after infusion with platelet-aggregating doses of 4 to 40 x 10(9) cells of *S. sanguis* 133-79. Infusion resulted in dose-dependent changes in electrocardiograms, blood pressure, heart rate, and cardiac contractility. These changes were consistent with the occurrence of MI. Platelets isolated from hyperlipidemic rabbits showed an accelerated *in vitro* aggregation response to strain 133-79. Cultured from immunosuppressed children with septic shock and signs of disseminated intravascular coagulation, more than 60% of isolates of viridans streptococci induced platelet aggregation when tested *in vitro*. The data are consistent with a thrombogenic role for *S. sanguis* in human disease, contributing to the development of the vegetative lesion in infective endocarditis and a thrombotic mechanism to explain the additional contributed risk of periodontitis to MI.

From: *Journal of Periodontology* 1996 October; Volume 67, Number 10, Supplement, pp. 1138-1142.

Article Title:
Periodontal disease as a risk factor for heart disease.

Loesche WJ.

School of Medicine, University of Michigan, Ann Arbor.

ABSTRACT: Many individuals with cardiovascular disease appear from epidemiologic studies to have either periodontal disease or to be edentulous. A Finnish group has provided evidence that after conventional risk factors for stroke and heart attacks have been accounted for, there still remains a significant relationship between dental disease and cardiovascular disease. A preliminary analysis of our own investigation of the interrelationship of medical and dental health shows that individuals with a high dental morbidity (i.e., edentulous or with many missing teeth) have a high prevalence of coronary heart disease and stroke. A model based on how smoking can predispose to periodontal disease is used to explain how periodontal disease could be a potential risk factor for heart disease.

From: *Compendium* 1994 August; Volume 15, Number 8, pp. 976, 978-982, 985-986.

Article Title:
Dental infections as a risk factor for acute myocardial infarction.

Mattila KJ.

First Department of Medicine, Helsinki University Central Hospital, Finland.

ABSTRACT: The so-called classic risk factors of coronary heart disease (CHD) do not explain all its clinical and epidemiological features. Recent evidence suggests that certain infections, among them dental infections, are involved in the pathogenesis of CHD. Case-control studies have revealed an association between dental infections and acute myocardial infarction and chronic coronary heart disease. A large epidemiological survey revealed an association between missing teeth and CHD and a recent 14-year follow-up of 9760 individuals showed that periodontitis is associated with an increased risk of coronary heart disease. Preliminary results suggest that the severity of dental infections correlates with the extent of coronary atheromatosis. Individuals with severe dental infections also have higher levels of von Willebrand factor antigen, leukocytes and fibrinogen. *Streptococcus sanguis* has been shown to aggregate human platelets *in vitro*. The mechanism behind the association between dental infections and CHD could be the effect of bacteria on the cells taking part in the pathogenesis of atherosclerosis and arterial thrombosis.

From: *European Heart Journal* 1993 December; Volume 14, Supplement K, pp. 51-53.

Article Title:
Chronic infections and the risk of carotid atherosclerosis: prospective results from a large population study.

Kiechl S, Egger G, Mayr M, Wiedermann CJ, Bonora E, Oberhollenzer F, Muggeo M, Xu Q, Wick G, Poewe W, Willeit J.

Departments of Neurology, University Clinic Innsbruck,

Innsbruck, Austria.

ABSTRACT: Chronic infections have been implicated in the pathogenesis of atherosclerosis, yet from an epidemiological perspective, this concept remains controversial. METHODS AND RESULTS: The Bruneck Study is a prospective population-based survey on the pathogenesis of atherosclerosis. In 826 men and women 40 to 79 years old (1990 baseline), 5-year changes in carotid atherosclerosis were thoroughly assessed by high-resolution duplex scanning. The presence of chronic respiratory, urinary tract, dental, and other infections was ascertained by standard diagnostic criteria. Chronic infections amplified the risk of atherosclerosis development in the carotid arteries. The association was most pronounced in subjects free of carotid atherosclerosis at baseline (age-/sex-adjusted odds ratio [95% CI] for any chronic infection versus none, 4.08 [2.42 to 6.85]; P:<0.0001) and applied to all types of chronic (bacterial) infections. It remained independently significant after adjustment for classic vascular risk attributes and extended to low-risk individuals free of conventional risk factors. Among subjects with chronic infections, atherosclerosis risk was highest in those with a prominent inflammatory response. Markers of systemic inflammation, such as soluble adhesion molecules and circulating bacterial endotoxin, and levels of soluble human heat-shock protein 60 and antibodies to mycobacterial heat-shock protein 65 were elevated in subjects with chronic infections and predictive of an increased risk of atherosclerosis. CONCLUSIONS: The present study provides solid evidence for a role of common chronic infections in human atherogenesis. Induction of systemic inflammation and autoimmunity may be potential pathophysiological links.

From: *Circulation* 2001 February; Volume 103, Number 8, pp. 1064-1070.

Article Title:
Dental infections in association with cerebral infarction in young and middle-aged men.

Syrjanen J, Peltola J, Valtonen V, Iivanainen M, Kaste M, Huttunen JK.

Department of Bacteriology and Immunology, University of Helsinki, Finland.

ABSTRACT: The association between dental infections and cerebral infarction was investigated in a case-control study involving 40 patients with ischaemic cerebral infarction under the age of 50, and 40 randomly selected community controls matched for sex and age. Poor oral health, as assessed by two indices measuring the severity of infections of teeth and periodontium, or by the presence of subgingival calculus or the presence of suppuration in the gingival pockets, was more common in male patients than in male controls, but no difference was observed in females. If severe dental infections were combined with other probable bacterial infections there were altogether 16 patients (40%) but only two controls (5%) who had suffered from a probable bacterial infection within 1 month or at the time of the stroke or when examined as a control (P less than 0.01). Our results suggest an association between bacterial infection and ischaemic cerebrovascular disease in patients under 50 years of age. Severe chronic dental infection seems to be an important type of infection associated with cerebral infarction in males.

From: *Journal of Internal Medicine* 1989 March; Volume 225, Number 3, pp. 179-184.

Article Title:
Dental disease: a frequently unrecognized cause of maxillary sinus abnormalities?

Abrahams JJ, Glassberg RM.

Department of Diagnostic Radiology, Yale University School of Medicine, New Haven, CT 06520-8042, USA.

ABSTRACT: Periodontal disease may be a frequently unrecognized cause of maxillary sinus disease. The purposes of this study were to determine if maxillary sinus disease is more prevalent in patients with periodontal disease than in an age-and-sex-matched control group and to show radiographically an association of focal maxillary sinus disease with periodontal disease. MATERIALS AND METHODS: Maxillary DentaScans (General Electric Medical Systems, Milwaukee, WI) of 84 patients (168 maxillary sinuses) with periodontal disease were retrospectively evaluated for the simple presence or absence of maxillary sinus disease. This group was compared with an age-and-sex-matched control population of 84 patients who were referred for head or neck CT scans in which the maxillary sinuses (including their inferior aspects) were visualized. For the likelihood of sinus disease in patients compared with controls, an odds ratio and a 95% confidence interval were calculated using the SYSTAT version 5.2 (SYSTAT, Evanston, IL). In the second portion of the study, the subject population alone was graded in the following fashion to establish a causal relationship: grade 0, no sinus disease; grade 1, focal sinus disease not adjacent to periodontal disease (unlikely to be caused by periodontal disease); grade 2, nonfocal sinus disease (complete opacification, air-fluid levels, or diffuse mucoperiosteal thickening; indeterminate cause), and grade 3, focal sinus disease adjacent to periodontal disease (likely to be caused by peri-

odontal disease). RESULTS: In the subject population—patients with periodontal disease who were referred for DentaScans—100 of 168 (60%) sinuses had sinus disease; in the control population, only 49 of 168 (29%) sinuses had sinus disease. The odds ratio for maxillary sinus disease in the patient population compared with controls was 3.6 (95% confidence interval, 2.3-5.6; p<.0001). The grading results of the subject population in the second portion of the study were grade 0, 68 sinuses (41%); grade 1, four sinuses (2%); grade 2, 32 sinuses (19%); and grade 3, 64 sinuses (38%). CONCLUSION: We have demonstrated a twofold increase in maxillary sinus disease in patients with periodontal disease and have shown a causal relationship. Recognition of this relationship may have an impact on the clinical management of patients, particularly those planning implant surgery.
From: *AJR. American Journal of Roentgenology* 1996 May; Volume 166, Number 5, pp. 1219-1223.

Article Title:
Relationships between chronic oral infectious diseases and systemic diseases.

Okuda K, Ebihara Y.
Oral Health Science Center, Tokyo Dental College, Chiba, Japan.

ABSTRACT: There are over 300 species of bacteria forming populations of several hundred billion in the human oral cavity. The number of bacteria reaches a thousand billion when the mouth is not sufficiently cleaned. Using saliva and gingival crevicular fluid as their main nutrients, these bacteria create their ecological niches on tooth surfaces, gingival crevices, saliva, dorsum linguae, and buccal and pharyngeal mucosa, threatening oral and systemic health. It is known that primary lesions of these chronic bacterial infections secondarily cause nephritis, rheumatoid arthritis, and dermatitis. Further, it has been demonstrated in recent years that bacteria inhabiting the oral cavity can cause bacterial pneumonia and endocarditis and that the periodontal disease-associated bacteria become causative agents for pregnancy troubles and are involved in blood circulation problems and coronary heart disease. Dentistry reviewed the theme of World Health Day, Oral Health for a Healthy Life, in 1994. The 8020 campaign to promote tooth care is also becoming established in Japan; however, the authors emphasized that this achievement is not the goal of dental health care. In this article, we explain the bases supporting the concept that oral health care, primarily mouth cleaning, is important for not only oral disease but also a healthy life.

From: *The Bulletin of Tokyo Dental College* 1998 August; Volume 39, Number 3, pp. 165-174.

Article Title:
Periodontal disease and risk of cerebrovascular disease: the first national health and nutrition examination survey and its follow-up study.

Wu T, Trevisan M, Genco RJ, Dorn JP, Falkner KL, Sempos CT.

Department of Social and Preventive Medicine, State University of New York at Buffalo, 3435 Main St, Buffalo, NY 14214.

ABSTRACT: Periodontal disease has been found to be a potential risk factor for coronary heart disease. However, its association with cerebrovascular accidents (CVAs) is much less studied. METHODS: This study examines the association between periodontal disease and CVA. The study cohort comprises 9962 adults aged 25 to 74 years who participated in the First National Health and Nutrition Examination Survey and its followup study. Baseline periodontal status was categorized into (1) no periodontal disease, (2) gingivitis, (3) periodontitis, and (4) edentulousness. All CVAs (International Classification of Diseases, Ninth Revision [ICD-9], codes 430-438) were ascertained by hospital records for nonfatal events and death certificates for fatal events. The first CVA, nonfatal or fatal, was used to define incidence. Relative risks were estimated by hazard ratios from the Cox proportional hazard model with adjustment for several demographic variables and well-established cardiovascular risk factors. Weights were used to generate risk estimates. RESULTS: Periodontitis is a significant risk factor for total CVA and, in particular, nonhemorrhagic stroke (ICD-9, 433-434 and 436-438). Compared with no periodontal disease, the relative risks (95% confidence intervals) for incident nonhemorrhagic stroke were 1.24 (0.74-2.08) for gingivitis, 2.11 (1.30-3.42) for periodontitis, and 1.41 (0.96-2.06) for edentulousness. For total CVA, the results were 1.02 (0.70-1.48) for gingivitis, 1.66 (1.15-2.39) for periodontitis, and 1.23 (0.91-1.66) for edentulousness. Increased relative risks for total CVA and nonhemorrhagic stroke associated with periodontitis were also seen in white men, white women, and African Americans. Similar results were found for fatal CVA. CONCLUSION: Periodontal disease is an important risk factor for total CVA and, in particular, nonhemorrhagic stroke.

From: *Archives of Internal Medicine* 2000 October; Volume 160, Number 18, pp. 2749-2755.

Article Title:
Association of the oral flora with important medical diseases.

Loesche WJ.

University of Michigan School of Dentistry, Department of Biologic and Material Sciences, Ann Arbor 48109, USA.

ABSTRACT: Recently, there have been case-control and epidemiologic investigations that strongly associate poor dental health with cardiovascular disease, preterm low birth weight infants, and early death from any cause. In a 7-year prospective study, dental disease was a significant predictor of coronary events leading to death after controlling for known coronary disease risk factors. Missing teeth displaces smoking as a risk factor for ischemic heart disease in another study. Periodontal disease was seven times more likely to be associated with a preterm delivery of a low birth weight infant than mother's age, race, number of live births, and use of tobacco or alcohol. This review examines the role of asymptomatic bacteremia as possibly explaining these associations, focusing on the bacterial load on the teeth as mediated via oral hygiene.

From: *Current Opinion in Periodontology* 1997, Volume 4, pp. 21-28.

Article Title:
Systemic diseases caused by oral microorganisms.

Debelian GJ, Olsen I, Tronstad L.

Division of Endodontics, University of Oslo, Norway.

ABSTRACT: Human endodontic and periodontal infections are associated with complex microfloras in which approximately 150, (in apical periodontitis) and 350 (in marginal periodontitis) bacterial species have been encountered. These infections are predominantly anaerobic, with gram-negative rods being the most common isolates. The anatomic closeness of this microflora to the bloodstream can facilitate bacteremia and systemic spread of bacterial by-products and immunocomplexes. A variety of clinical procedures such as tooth extraction, periodontal and endodontic treatment, may cause translocation of microorganisms from the oral cavity to the bloodstream. The microorganisms that gain entrance to the blood circulate throughout the body, but are usually eliminated by the host (reticuloendothelial system) within minutes. However, in patients with ineffective heart valves or vascular diseases, bacteremia can be a potential danger, leading most commonly to infective endocarditis and myocardial or cerebral infarction. Other forms of systemic diseases such as brain abscesses, hematological infections and implant infections have also been related to oral microorganisms.

From: *Endodontics & Dental Traumatology* 1994 April; Volume 10, Number 2, pp. 57-65.

Article Title:
Systemic dissemination as a result of oral infection in individuals 50 years of age and older.

Navazesh M, Mulligan R.

Department of Dental Medicine & Public Health, University of Southern California, School of Dentistry, Los Angeles 90089-0641, USA.

ABSTRACT: The oral pathosis caused by systemic disorders in middle-aged and elderly adults has been the focus of many publications in recent years. The intraoral soft and hard tissue changes associated with systemic disorders, medications, chemotherapy, and radiation treatment have been well-investigated and-documented. Far less attention has been paid to the role of oral infection as the etiology of systemic disorders. A literature review (1980-1994) is provided here focusing on well-documented cases in which systemic disorders were caused by oral foci of infections. This paper attempts to raise the level of awareness of practitioners in considering possible systemic complications caused by oral infection. It also emphasizes the need for further longitudinal studies in this field involving healthy and medically compromised elderly individuals.

From: *Special Care in Dentistry* 1995 January-February; Volume 15, Number 1, pp. 11-19.

Article Title:
Dental infections and atherosclerosis.

Beck JD, Pankow J, Tyroler HA, Offenbacher S.

Department of Dental Ecology, Center for Oral and Systemic Disease, University of North Carolina at Chapel Hill, USA.

ABSTRACT: In most countries, coronary heart disease is one of the leading causes of morbidity and death. This report reviews the current evidence indicating that oral conditions (specifically periodontitis) may be a risk factor for atherosclerosis and its clinical manifestations and provides new preliminary data. This review is done in the context of the research indicating that inflammation plays a central role in atherogenesis and that there is a substantial systemic microbial and inflammatory burden associated with periodontal disease. Our review concentrates on 5 longitudinal studies that show oral conditions being associated with the onset of coronary heart disease while controlling for a variety of established coronary heart disease risk factors. In addition to published evidence, preliminary findings from our Dental Atherosclerosis Risk in Communities study also indicate that periodontal disease is associated with carotid intimal-medial wall thickness, a measure of subclinical atherosclerosis, adjusting for factors known to be associated with both conditions.

From: *American Heart Journal* 1999 November; Volume 138, Number 5 Pt 2, pp. S528-S533.

Article Title:
Potential pathogenic mechanisms of periodontitis associated pregnancy complications.

Offenbacher S, Jared HL, O'Reilly PG, Wells SR, Salvi GE, Lawrence HP, Socransky SS, Beck JD.

University of North Carolina at Chapel Hill, School of Dentistry, Department of Periodontology, USA.

ABSTRACT: During normal pregnancy, maternal hormones and locally acting cytokines play a key role in regulating the onset of labor, cervical ripening, uterine contraction, and delivery. Maternal infections during pregnancy have been demonstrated to perturb this normal cytokine and hormone-regulated gestation, sometimes resulting in preterm labor, preterm premature rupture of membranes, and preterm low birth weight (PLBW), i.e., < 2,500 g and < 37 weeks of gestation. Our research focus has been to determine whether periodontal infections can provide sufficient challenge to the mother to trigger PLBW. New experiments from 48 case-control subjects have measured gingival crevicular fluid (GCF) levels of PGE(2) and IL-1-beta to determine whether mediator levels were related to current pregnancy outcome. In addition, the levels of 4 periodontal pathogens were measured by using microbe-specific DNA probes. Results indicate that GCF-PGE(2) levels are significantly higher in PLBW mothers, as compared with normal birth weight (NBW) controls (131.4 +/-21.8 vs. 62.6 +/-10.3 [mean +/-SE ng/mL], respectively, at P = 0.02). Furthermore, within primiparous PLBW mothers, there was a significant inverse association between birth weight (as well as gestational age) and GCF-PGE(2) levels at P = 0.023. These data suggest a dose-response relationship for increasing GCF-PGE(2) as a marker of current periodontal disease activity and decreasing birth weight. Microbial data indicate that 4 organisms associated with mature plaque and progressing periodontitis—*Bacteroides forsythus*, *Porphyromonas gingivalis*, *Actinobacillus actinomycetemcomitans*, and *Treponema denticola*—were detected at higher levels in PLBW mothers, as compared to NBW controls. These data suggest that biochemical measures of maternal periodontal status and oral microbial burden are associated with current PLBW.

From: *Annals of Periodontology* 1998 July; Volume 3, Number 1, pp. 233-250.

Article Title:
Poor periodontal health of the pregnant woman as a risk factor for low birth weight.

Dasanayake AP.

Department of Oral Biology, School of Dentistry, University of Alabama at Birmingham. USA.

ABSTRACT: In both developed and developing countries, low birth weight (LBW) has a tremendous impact on both the health care system and the individual families affected. This warrants the continuous search for risk factors for LBW that are amenable to prevention. Can poor oral health of the pregnant woman be one such factor? In a 1:1 matched case-control study (N = 55 pairs), we evaluated the hypothesis that poor oral health of the pregnant woman is a risk factor for LBW. The effect of periodontal and dental caries status of the woman at the time of delivery on the birth weight of the infant was evaluated by using conditional logistic regression analyses, while controlling for known risk factors for LBW. Mothers of LBW infants were shorter, less educated, married to men of lower occupational class, had less healthy areas of gingiva and more areas with bleeding and calculus, and gained less weight during the pregnancy. Conditional logistic regression analyses indicated that mothers with more healthy areas of gingiva (OR = 0.3, 95% CI = 0.12—0.72) and those who were taller (OR = 0.86, 95% CI = 0.75—0.98) had a lower risk of giving birth to an LBW infant. Risk of LBW was higher in mothers who had no or late prenatal care (OR = 3.9, 95% CI = 1.24—12.2). We conclude that poor periodontal health of the mother is a potential independent risk factor for LBW.

From: *Annals of Periodontology* 1998 July; Volume 3, Number 1, pp. 206-212.

Article Title:
Germs, Dr. Billings, and the theory of focal infection.

Gibbons RV.

Department of Medicine, Madigan Army Medical Center, Tacoma, Washington 98499-5000, USA.

ABSTRACT: Our understanding of infectious diseases continues to expand rapidly, and has led to the realization that microorganisms are responsible for, or at least contribute to, numerous diseases that were never before associated with infectious etiologies. However, a review of medical history reminds us that this is not so novel an idea. Not long after the widespread acceptance of bacteriology and the germ theory and with an increased awareness of public hygiene, there was a period during which it seemed that nearly all diseases would prove to be the result of infections. One popular proposal that championed such an idea was the theory of focal infection. This article reviews this theory by considering the key concepts and developments that likely inspired it, and examines the work of the theory's most visible proponent, Dr. Frank Billings.

From: *Clinical Infectious Diseases* 1998 September; Volume 27, Number 3, pp. 627-633.

Article Title:
Brain abcess following dental infection.

Henig EF, Derschowitz T, Shalit M, Toledo E, Tikva P, Aviv T.

ABSTRACT: A 48-year-old woman underwent root canal treatment of the upper left lateral incisor and lower right second premolar. Close to the conclusion of the endodontic treatment she complained about headaches. Later on, because of aggravation of her condition, with headaches, fever, malaise, weakness, and numbness of the right limbs, she was admitted to the hospital. The disease progressed to an epileptic state, with appearance of a right hemiparesis. A brain scan and carotid arteriogram revealed the presence of a mass occupying the left parietal space. Craniotomy disclosed an abscess containing yellow pus from which *Streptococcus viridans* was cultured. After thorough surgical cleansing of the area, removal of the bone for decompression, and treatment with ampicillin the patient improved gradually and slowly regained the mobility of her right side.

From: *Oral Surgery, Oral Medicine, and Oral Pathology* 1978 June; Volume 45, Number 6, pp. 955-958.

II. CAVITATION ARTICLES

Article Title:
Neuralgia-inducing cavitational osteonecrosis (NICO). Osteomyelitis in 224 jawbone samples from patients with facial neuralgia.

Bouquot JE, Roberts AM, Person P, Christian J.

Department of Oral Surgery, West Virginia University School of Dentistry.

ABSTRACT: A somewhat obscure etiologic theory for facial neuralgias presumes a low-grade osteomyelitis of the jaws that produces neural degeneration with subsequent production of inappropriate pain signals. Animal investigations and treatment successes with human patients based on this theory lend it credence. The present study examined 224 tissue samples removed from alveolar bone cavities in 135 patients with trigeminal neuralgia or atypical facial neuralgia. All tissue samples demonstrated clear evidence of chronic intraosseous inflammation. The most common microscopic features included dense marrow fibrosis or "scar" formation, a sprinkling of lymphocytes in a relative absence of other inflammatory cells (especially histiocytes), and smudged, nonresorbing necrotic bone flakes. Very little healing or new bone formation was visible. These lesions were able to burrow several centimeters to initiate distant cavities. The present preliminary investigation cannot prove etiology, but the presence of intraosseous inflammation in every single jawbone specimen in these patients and certain clinical and treatment aspects of these lesions (to be reported later) has led the authors to recommend the term neuralgia-inducing cavitational osteonecrosis or NICO for these lesions.

From: *Oral Surgery, Oral Medicine, and Oral Pathology* 1992 March; Volume 73, Number 3, pp. 307-319.

Article Title:
Chronic mandibular osteomyelitis.

Harris LF.

ABSTRACT: Chronic osteomyelitis of the mandible is an infrequently reported condition, but recent experience with six cases over a 14-month period suggests it is more common than appreciated. Chronic mandibular osteomyelitis results from odontogenic infection, postextraction complication, trauma, or irradiation to the mandible. Clinical findings include local pain and swelling and trismus, but constitutional symptoms are unusual. Radiologic examination discloses radiolucent areas, bony destruction, and sequestrum formation. Pathogenic organisms are normal oral flora, *Staphylococcus aureus*, and aerobic gram-negative bacilli. Chronic mandibular osteomyelitis must be differentiated from malignant disease involving the mandible. Diagnosis is accomplished by bone biopsy and culture. Treatment involves through surgical debridement and prolonged antimicrobial therapy. Osteoradionecrosis of the mandible is extremely recalcitrant to conventional therapy, but aggressive surgery and treatment have proven effective.

From: *Southern Medical Journal* 1986 June; Volume 79, Number 6, pp. 696-697.
Article Title:

Infectious foci in chronic osteomyelitis of the jaws.

Wannfors K, Hammarstrom L.

ABSTRACT: Chronic osteomyelitis of the jaws has a varied clinical appearance and an unclear etiology. In a retrospective study based on case histories and histological material from 24 patients with chronic osteomyelitis, no specific correlation could be found between clinical symptoms and morphological changes in bone. In 10 patients, bacteria were found in certain foci such as osteocytic lacunae of necrotic bone and dentinal tubules of embedded tooth fragments. In these foci, the bacteria probably escaped the immunological response as well as the antibiotic treatment. From these foci, the bacteria might maintain an inflammatory reaction in the surrounding bone. In some patients, the mandibular canal seemed to be a pathway for the spreading of the inflammatory process.

From: *International Journal of Oral Surgery* 1985 December; Volume 14, Number 6, pp. 493-503.

Article Title:
Trigeminal neuralgia—a new treatment concept.

Shaber EP, Krol AJ.

ABSTRACT: A concept for the treatment of trigeminal neuralgia is presented. On the basis of distinctive pain patterns, localized areas of pathosis within the jawbones are detected and obliterated. To date, we have treated eight patients with idiopathic trigeminal neuralgia. All patients have experienced total or near total abatement of pain.

From: *Oral Surgery, Oral Medicine, and Oral Pathology* 1980

April; Volume 49, Number 4, pp. 286-293.

Article Title:
Jawbone cavities and trigeminal and atypical facial neuralgias.

Ratner EJ, Person P, Kleinman DJ, Shklar G, Socransky SS.

ABSTRACT: The possible role of dental and oral disease in the etiology of idiopathic trigeminal and atypical facial neuralgias has been examined. Among thirty-eight patients with idiopathic trigeminal neuralgia and twenty-three patients with atypical facial neuralgia, there was in nearly all instances a close relationship between pain experienced and the existence of cavities in alveolar bone and jawbone of the patients. The cavities were at the sites of previous tooth extractions and, although at times more than 1 cm. in a given diameter, were usually not detectable by x-rays. A new method for their detection and localization was developed empirically, based on the observation that peripheral infiltration of local anesthetic into or very close to the bone cavity rapidly abolished trigger and pain perception by patients during persistence of the anesthetic action. Histopathologic examination of bone removed from cavities by curettage revealed, in both idiopathic trigeminal and atypical facial neuralgias, a similar pattern characterized by a highly vascular abnormal healing response of bone. Some lesions presented a mild chronic inflammatory (lymphocytic) infiltration. Preliminary microbiologic studies of material from the walls of the cavities showed the existence within them of a complex, mixed polymicrobial aerobic and anaerobic flora. Treatment consisted of vigorous curettage of the bone cavities, repeated if necessary, plus administration of antibiotics to induce healing and filling-in of the cavities by new bone. Responses of patients to the above treatment consisted of marked to complete pain remissions, the longest of which has been for 9 years. Complete healing leads to complete and persistent pain remissions. It was concluded that in both idiopathic trigeminal and atypical facial neuralgias, dental and oral pathoses may be major etiologic factors.

From: *Oral Surgery, Oral Medicine, and Oral Pathology* 1979 July; Volume 48, Number 1, pp. 3-20.

Article Title:
Osteomyelitis of the jaws.

Rangne A, Ruud A.

ABSTRACT: Material consisting of 16 patients examined and/or treated under the diagnosis osteomyelitis is reported. A description is given of the history, etiology, clinical and radiographic findings, results of histologic and microbiologic examinations, blood chemistry, diagnostic subgroups, findings at operation and the surgical and antibiotic therapy used. The results of treatment at short-term follow-up are given. Of nine patients observed 5 months or longer, six showed signs of healing, while the result was judged as uncertain in two cases and unsuccessful in one.

From: *International Journal of Oral Surgery* 1978 December; Volume 7, Number 6, pp. 523-527.

Article Title:
[Osteomyelitis of the jaw.]

[Article in German]

Neumann VH, Steinbrecher G, Thimann I.

ABSTRACT: A brief description of nomenclature differences and classification principles is followed by a report of the results from an analysis of cases of osteomyelitis of the jaw, which have been treated during the years 1967-1972. During this period, altogether 745 patients with soft-tissue infection and 72 patients with osteomyelitis have been treated at the clinic. The chronic form of osteomyelitis is considerably more frequent than the acute one. The odontogenic mode of infection prevails by far. The flora of causative organisms and the resistance conditions are dealt with separately. The mixed flora dominates; monoinfections are rare. Antibiotherapy occupies the first place in the treatment of the acute forms whereas surgical intervention is the method of choice in the treatment of the chronic forms of osteomyelitis.

From: *Stomatologie der DDR* 1975 January; Volume 25, Number 1, pp. 31-34.

Article Title:
[Clinics and therapy of the osteomyelitis of the lower jaw.]

[Article in German]

Schelhorn P, Zenk W.

ABSTRACT: During the last three decades the clinical picture of osteomyelitis has considerably changed. Acute cases have become rarer than in the past. The outbreak of the disease to be observed in recent times is primarily of a subacute chronic stage. These non-characteristic symptoms make diagnosis more difficult. Acute cases of osteomyelitis are treated with antibiotics; chronic cases should surgically be approached as early as possible. Surgical methods used are above all decortication as well as transplantation of autogenous spongiosa.

From: *Stomatologie der DDR* 1989 October; Volume 39, Number 10, pp. 672-676.

Article Title:
Blood flow in jaw bones affected by chronic osteomyelitis.

Wannfors K, Gazelius B.
Department of Oral Pathology, School of Dentistry, Huddinge, Sweden.

ABSTRACT: In order to study circulatory changes throughout the course of chronic osteomyelitis of the jaws, blood flow in bone affected by osteomyelitis was assessed in 14 patients, by means of laser Doppler flowmetry (LDF). The difference in perfusion between the osteomyelitic bone and corresponding sites on the opposite healthy jaw was evaluated. The patients were classified into two groups according to the clinical activity of their disease. A significantly reduced bone blood flow was recorded in the jaw during non-active stages, while an increased flow was associated with the initial stage of disease and the inflammatory exacerbations. No pre-existing vascular disorders were discovered prior to the development of this disease. However, a long-standing local inflammation of the jaw bone was associated with a persistent reduction in blood flow. In 12 healthy subjects, blood flow in the left jaw was found not to be statistically different to that in the right jaw.

From: *The British Journal of Oral & Maxillofacial Surgery* 1991 June; Volume 29, Number 3, pp. 147-153.

Article Title:
Cavitational bone defect: a diagnostic challenge.

Segall RO, del Rio CE.

Department of Endodontics, The University of Texas Health Science Center at San Antonio.

ABSTRACT: A patient with a history of trauma to the maxillary left anterior region presented with chronic pain of unknown etiology. Root canal therapy and periradicular surgery failed to resolve the persistent pain. A second surgical procedure revealed a bone cavity superior and distopalatally to the apex of the maxillary left lateral incisor. The suspected etiology was necrotic bone removed from the bone cavity.

From: *Journal of Endodontics* 1991 August; Volume 17, Number 8, pp. 396-400.

Article Title:
Osteomyelitis of the jaws: a 50-year perspective.

Hudson JW.

Department of Oral Maxillofacial Surgery, University of Tennessee Medical Center, Knoxville.
ABSTRACT: The incidence of osteomyelitis of the jaws has decreased dramatically, except for a few subsets of individuals. This has been due, in no small part, to the availability of bacteriocidal antimicrobial therapy. The pathogenesis of osteomyelitis of the jaws is predominately due to odontogenic microorganisms rather than the classic skin contaminant, *Staphylococcus*. This causative relationship relegates the classifi-

cation of osteomyelitis of the bimaxillary skeleton to predominately that of contiguous foci. These may be regionally progressive, secondary to microvascular compromise brought about by inherent flaws in regional anatomic calcified tissue vascular perfusion as well as by inflammatory metaplastic processes. Diagnosis is based on the presence of painful sequestra and suppurative areas of tooth-bearing jaw bone unresponsive to debridement and conservative therapy. This is usually accompanied by regional or systemic compromise of the immune response, microvascular decompensation, or both. Treatment of both acute and chronic forms of the disease is successful if surgically supported. Sustained bacteriocidal antibiotic therapy is pertinent, especially in the face of potentially refractory virulent microorganisms and compromised regional vascular penetrance. The use of adjunctive hyperbaric oxygen therapy also may be included in the more refractory forms of osteomyelitis of the jaws to enhance the local and regional immune response of the jaws as well as to produce microvascular neoangiogenesis for reperfusion support. With resolution of infection, hard and soft tissue reconstruction may be necessary to augment the reparative process.

From: *Journal of Oral and Maxillofacial Surgery* 1993 December; Volume 51, Number 12, pp. 1294-1301.

Article Title:
[Chronic osteomyelitis of mandibulae]

[Article in Japanese]

Sasaki J, Nameta K.

Department of Oral Surgery, Tokaki University School of Medicine.

ABSTRACT: As the human lower jaw (mandibula) itself is a hard bone, and when bacterial inflammation occurs in it by pericoronal infection of the 3rd molar or apical infection of caries tooth, the inflammation remains in the bone marrow and often progresses to acute osteomyelitis. The prominent sign of acute osteomyelitis in the lower jaw is mental nerve palsy, which is the so-called Vincent's Syndrome. The causative organisms are not different from those of the common odontogenic infections. Recently, we have identified some strains of Oral Streptococci tolerant against PCs and Cefems and also ones capable of biofilm formation. When antimicrobial agents or drainage proves unsuccessful, acute osteomyelitis may become chronic, which is more difficult to treat. Surgical procedures, such as, debridement or decortication of cortex bone, are necessary in most cases. If these surgical procedures do not give satisfactory results, the amputation of the jaw is not rare.
From: *Nippon Rinsho. Japanese Journal of Clinical Medicine* 1994 February; Volume 52, Number 2, pp. 507-511.

Article Title:
Osteomyelitis of the jaws.

Bernier S, Clermont S, Maranda G, Turcotte JY.

Sir Mortimer B. Davis Jewish General Hospital, Montreal.

ABSTRACT: Osteomyelitis is described as an inflammation of bone and bone marrow that may develop in the jaws following a chronic odontogenic infection or for a variety of other reasons. This situation may be acute, sub-acute or chronic, resulting in a totally different clinical picture.

From: *Journal of the Canadian Dental Association* 1995 May;

Volume 61, Number 5, pp. 441-442, 445-448.

Article Title:
Aureobasidium **infection of the jaw.**

Koppang HS, Olsen I, Stuge U, Sandven P.

Department of Oral Pathology, University of Oslo, Norway.

ABSTRACT: A 32-yr-old white North American male resident of Norway presented with an asymptomatic radiolucency first identified 3 yr after the removal of an impacted mandibular right third molar in Southern California 16 yr previously. Surgical exploration revealed an intraosseous cavity filled with a black, homogeneous, gelatinous substance thought to be foreign material, but which was diagnosed histologically as containing black yeasts. Cultivation of a microbiologic sample for 6 wk grew black yeast-like colonies. The yeast isolate was identified as an *Aureobasidium* species different from the typical *A. pullulans*. A blood sample was negative with regard to antibodies both with double diffusion technique and ELISA. Also, examination with respect to dermatologic manifestations gave negative results. Flucytocin 10 g/d was administered systemically for 30 d. Six months postoperatively bone regeneration was satisfactory radiologically.

From: *Journal of Oral Pathology & Medicine* 1991 April; Volume 20, Number 4, pp. 191-195.

Article Title:
Heterozygosity for the Leiden mutation of the factor V gene, a common pathoetiology for osteonecrosis of the jaw, with thrombophilia augmented by exogenous estrogens.

Glueck CJ, McMahon RE, Bouquot JE, Triplett D, Gruppo R, Wang P.

Cholesterol Center, Jewish Hospital, Cincinnati, OH 45229, USA.

ABSTRACT: We assessed whether heterozygosity for the thrombophilic Leiden mutation of the factor V gene (MFV) was pathogenetic for alveolar osteonecrosis of the jaw and chronic facial pain (neuralgia-inducing cavitational osteonecrosis (NICO)) in 89 patients with NICO. A second specific aim was to assess for thrombophilic synergism between exogenous estrogens and MFV for development of osteonecrosis of the jaw. MFV was found in 24% of the patients, 16 (21%) of 76 women and 5 (39%) of 13 men. The mutation was much less common in healthy normal controls: 3 (3%) of 101 women (chi2 = 14.8, p = 0.001) and 4 (3.7%) of 108 men (chi2 = 20.4, p = 0.001). Patients with and without MFV did not differ in tissue plasminogen activator activity, plasminogen activator inhibitor activity, proteins C and S, lipoprotein (a), or anticardiolipin antibodies (p > 0.05). Use of standard-dose oral contraceptives and/or postmenopausal estrogens before the development of NICO was more common in female patients with MFV (13 (81%) of 16) than in those without it (23 (38%) of 60; chi2 = 9.33, p = 0.002). When the thrombophilic effects of such exogenous estrogens were superimposed on the familial resistance to activated protein C associated with MFV, thrombophilia was augmented and the risk of osteonecrosis was increased. Since heterozygosity for this mutation occurs in at least 3% of unselected, healthy women, measurement of resistance to activated protein C and MFV would identify women at high risk for venous thrombosis and osteonecrosis, in whom use of oral contraceptives or postmenopausal estrogens might be contraindicated, while identifying a much larger group of women (approximately 97%) without the mutation whose risk from exogenous estrogens would be low.

From: *The Journal of Laboratory and Clinical Medicine* 1997 November; Volume 130, Number 5, pp. 540-543.

III. ARTICLES ON DENTAL TOXINS

Article Title:
Short-chain carboxylic acid concentration in human gingival crevicular fluid.

Niederman R, Buyle-Bodin Y, Lu BY, Robinson P, Naleway C.

Forsyth Dental Center, Boston, Massachusetts, USA.

ABSTRACT: Short-chain carboxylic acids (e.g., lactic acid, propionic acid, butyric acid) are metabolic by-products of bacterial metabolism, which can accumulate in the gingival crevice. It is of no small consequence, therefore, that 1-to 5-mM concentrations of these acids exhibit significant biological activity, including the ability to alter cell proliferation and gene expression in cells of importance to the periodontium. This communication reports on the *in vivo* concentrations of propionic and butyric acid in the gingival crevices of periodontal subjects with severe and mild disease. The results indicated that severely diseased subjects exhibited a > 10-fold increase in the mM concentration of these acids when compared with mildly diseased subjects (mean propionic acid-severe = 9.5 +/-1.8 mM, and mild = 0.8 +/-0.3 mM; mean butyric acid-severe = 2.6 +/-0.4 mM, and mild = 0.2 +/-0.04 mM). These differences (mean +/-SE) were significant ($p < 0.0001$). The propionic and butyric acid concentrations were below detection limits in healthy sites of mildly diseased subjects. The propionic and butyric acid concentrations also associated significantly with clinical measures of disease severity (e.g., pocket depth, attachment level) and inflammation (e.g., subgingival temperature, % of sites bleeding when probed), and with the total microbial load (all p < 0.05). Taken together, these data suggest that short-chain carboxylic acids play a mediating role in periodontal disease pathogenesis.

From: *Journal of Dental Research* 1997 January; Volume 76, Number 1, pp. 575-579.

Article Title:
The relationship of gingival crevicular fluid short chain carboxylic acid concentration to gingival inflammation.

Niederman R, Buyle-Bodin Y, Lu BY, Naleway C, Robinson P, Kent R.

Forsyth Dental Center, Boston, MA.

ABSTRACT: Short-chain carboxylic acids (SCCA; C < or = 5; e.g., lactic acid, propionic acid, butyric acid) are metabolic by-products of bacterial metabolism, which accumulate in the gingival crevice, and exhibit significant biological activity, including the ability to alter gene expression. It has been hypothesized that among the activities of SCCAs are their ability to contribute to gingival inflammation. This concept complements the notion that specific periodontal pathogens are the causative agents of gingival inflammation. To begin testing these 2 hypotheses, we examined the relationship between SCCA concentrations, specific putative periodontal pathogens, and gingival inflammation in medically healthy periodontally diseased subjects. We reasoned that if SCCAs and/or specific periodontal pathogens were causative gingival inflammatory agents, gingival inflammation should increase with increasing concentration of the inflammatory mediator. We also recognized that other clinical variables needed to be controlled for, and an objective quantitative assessment of gingival inflammation used. To accomplish these tasks, sites within subjects were stratified by location and pocket depth, and the following quantified: bacterial presence; SCCA concentration; and gingival inflammation. The results indicated that gingival inflammation directly and significantly correlated with SCCA concentrations in the maxillary and mandibular molars, incisors and canines (all $r >$ or $= 0.47$; all $p <$ or $= 0.015$; too few bicuspids were available for complete analysis). The relationship between gingival inflammation and SCCA concentration was best described by a natural log relationship. Gingival inflammation did not, however, correlate positively with either the total number of specific putative periodontal pathogens, or the sum of subsets of these pathogens ($-0.31 <$ or $= r <$ or $= 0.39$; $0.08 <$ or $= p <$ or $= 0.75$) for any of the locations. Finally, the SCCA concentration did not correlate with the level of individual or groups of pathogens. These data, together with historical work and other preliminary data, support the hypothesis that SCCA, rather than specific putative periodontal pathogens, may be a causative agent in gingival inflammation. This work may, in part, begin to explain the apparent lack of a direct relationship between current gingival inflammation and the prediction of bacterially mediated periodontal attachment loss.

From: *Journal of Clinical Periodontology* 1996 August; Volume 23, Number 8, pp. 743-749.

Article Title:
The formation of hydrogen sulfide and methyl mercaptan by oral bacteria.

Persson S, Edlund MB, Claesson R, Carlsson J.

Department of Oral Microbiology, University of Umiea, Sweden.

ABSTRACT: The capacity to form volatile sulfur compounds was tested in bacteria isolated from subgingival microbiotas and in a representative number of reference strains. A majority of the 75 tested oral bacterial species and 7 unnamed bacterial taxa formed significant amounts of hydrogen sulfide from L-cysteine. The most active bacteria were found in the genera *Peptostreptococcus, Eubacterium, Selenomonas, Centipeda, Bacteroides* and *Fusobacterium*. Methyl mercaptan from L-methionine was formed by some members of the genera *Fusobacterium, Bacteroides, Porphyromonas* and *Eubacterium*. When incubated in serum for 7 d, the most potent producers of hydrogen sulfide were *Treponema denticola* and the black-pigmented species, *Bacteroides intermedius, Bacteroides loescheii, Porphyromonas endodontalis* and *Porphyromonas gingivalis*. *P. endodontalis* and *P. gingivalis* also produced significant amounts of methyl mercaptan in serum. No other volatile sulfur compound was detected in serum or in the presence of L-cysteine and L-methionine. These findings significantly increase the list of oral bacteria known to produce volatile sulfur compounds.

From: *Oral Microbiology and Immunology* 1990 August; Volume 5, Number 4, pp. 195-201.

IV. ARTICLES EXAMINING SOURCES OF DENTAL INFECTION

Article Title:
Occurrence of invading bacteria in radicular dentin of periodontally diseased teeth: microbiological findings.

Giuliana G, Ammatuna P, Pizzo G, Capone F, D'Angelo M.

Department of Periodontology, University of Palermo, Italy.

ABSTRACT: Bacterial invasion in roots of periodontally diseased teeth, which has been recently documented using cultural and microscopic techniques, may be important in the pathogenesis of periodontal disease. The purpose of this investigation was to determine the occurrence and the species of invading bacteria in radicular dentin of periodontally diseased teeth. Samples were taken from the middle layer of radicular dentin of 26 periodontally diseased teeth. 14 healthy teeth were used as controls. Dentin samples were cultured anaerobically. The chosen methodology allowed the determination of the numbers of bacteria present in both deeper and outer part of dentinal tubules, and the bacterial concentration in dentin samples, expressed as colony forming units per mg of tissue (CFU/mg). Invading bacteria was detected in 14 (53.8%) samples from periodontally diseased teeth. The bacterial concentration ranged from 831.84 to 11971.3 CFU/mg (mean+/-standard deviation: 3043.15+/-2763.13). Microorganisms identified included putative periodontal pathogens such as *Prevotella intermedia*, *Porphyromonas gingivalis*, *Fusobacterium nucleatum*, *Bacteroides forsythus*, *Peptostreptococcus micros* and *Streptococcus intermedius*. These findings suggest that radicular dentin could act as bacterial reservoir from which periodontal pathogens can recolonize treated periodontal pockets, contributing to the failure of therapy and recurrence of disease.

From: *Journal of Clinical Periodontology* 1997 July; Volume 24, Number 7, pp. 478-485.

Article Title:
Anaerobic infections in the head and neck region.

Tabaqchali S.

Department of Medical Microbiology, St Bartholomew's Hospital, Medical College, West Smithfield, London, United Kingdom.

ABSTRACT: Anaerobic bacteria form the predominant flora of the oral cavity, outnumbering facultative organisms by 10-1,000: 1. The type of anaerobic bacteria and their concentration depend on the anatomical site and the degree of anaerobiosis in the different sites in the mouth. Three groups of anaerobic bacteria inhabit the oral cavity; the strict anaerobes, the moderate anaerobes, and the microaerophilic group of organisms. The majority of anaerobic bacterial infections occurring in the region of the mouth, head and neck are caused by the commensal flora. These infections include dental and periodontal disease where the predominant organisms are *Bacteroides* species, *Veillonella*, *Bifidobacteria*, *Peptococcus*, *Peptostreptococcus* and *Propionibacterium* species. More recently, *Bacteroides endontalis* has been isolated from a periapical abscess of endodontal origin and *B. gingivalis*, *B. intermedius*, *Haemophilus actinomycetemcomitans* and *Wollinella* species in chronic periodontal disease. *Treponema* species and other strict anaerobes are seen in smears of severe periodontal disease and acute necrotising gingivitis, but have not yet been isolated in pure culture. Until such time, their role in disease remains uncertain. Fusobacterium nucleatum is specially associated with severe orofacial infections, which may extend into the mediastinum. Other anaerobic infections include chronic otitis media, chronic sinusitis and mastoiditis, and brain abscess. Treatment of these conditions should include the use of beta-lactamase resistant antimicrobials, such as clindamycin or one of the nitroimidazoles with penicillin.

From: *Scandinavian Journal of Infectious Diseases. Supplementum* 1988; Volume 57, pp. 24-34.

Article Title:
Bacteriology of dental infections.

Asikainen S, Alaluusua S.

Department of Periodontology, University of Helsinki, Finland.

ABSTRACT: The most common dental diseases, periodontal disease and dental caries, are chronic infections caused by bacteria of normal oral flora. When these bacteria increase in number and irritation exceeds the host defence threshold, disease arises. The human oral flora comprises more than 300 different bacteria. During the last decade approximately 10 species, mainly Gram-negative anaerobes, have been noted as putative pathogens in periodontal disease. The Gram-positive and facultatively anaerobic mutans streptococci are aetiologically the most important bacteria in dental caries. Data have rapidly increased on the association of these bacteria with certain periodontal diseases or caries, on phenotypic and genotypic characteristics, pathogenic mechanisms, antibiotic susceptibility patterns and transmission among family members. Chronic dental infections have been the focus of renewed interest because of recent advances in oral microbiology as well as in medicine. We now know that in addition to oral streptococci, recently classified, fastidious periodontal anaerobes can be detected from various extra-oral infections. Oral bacteria may spread into the blood stream through ulcerated epithelium in diseased periodontal pockets and cause transient bacteraemias, which are regarded as increased risk, especially for immunocompromised patients or persons with endoprotheses. In these patients, routine antibiotic prophylaxis is recommended for invasive dental care procedures. Also the new association between dental infections and myocardial/cerebral infarction has offered new challenges for cooperation between dental and medical researchers.

From: *European Heart Journal* 1993 December; Volume 14, Supplement K, pp. 43-50.

V. ARTICLES DOCUMENTING THE CHRONIC INFECTIONS IN ROOT CANAL TREATED TEETH

Article Title:
Scanning electron microscopy of bacteria in the apical part of root canals in permanent teeth with periapical lesions.

Molven O, Olsen I, Kerekes K.

Department of Cardiology and Endodontics, School of Dentistry, University of Bergen, Norway.

ABSTRACT: The most apical 2 mm of the root canals of periapically diseased roots were examined for microorganisms by scanning electron microscopy (SEM). Bacteria in this area were observed in 10 out of 12 (83.3%) cases. The two remaining cases exhibited bacteria more coronally, with tissue remnants between the bacterial front and the apical foramen. Rod-shaped bacteria dominated, but filaments, spirochetes and cocci were also seen. Cocci and rods sometimes formed micro-colonies. Occasionally, cocci were seen attached to filaments forming "corn-cob"-like structures. Deposits resembling bacterial plaque were also found inside the root canal. SEM is useful for studying microbial topography of the apical root canal.

From: *Endodontics & Dental Traumatology* 1991 October; Volume 7, Number 5, pp. 226-229.

Article Title:
Similarities in the microfloras of root canals and deep periodontal pockets.

Kerekes K, Olsen I.

Dental Faculty, University of Oslo, Norway.

ABSTRACT: Although not universally accepted, retrospective histological, roentgenological and microbiological studies have indicated that cross-infection can occur between infected pulps and deep periodontal pockets. This review provides examples of similarities in the microfloras of these adjacent oral sites, supporting the idea that infection spreads from one site to the other. The organisms most often involved are probably *bacteroides*, *fusobacteria*, *eubacteria*, spirochetes, *wolinellas*, *selenomonas*, *campylobacter*, and *peptostreptococci*. Important qualities of cross-infecting organisms may be the ability to survive in highly reduced environments and motility. Precautions should be taken to prevent *in vivo* seeding of such microorganisms, particularly in compromised teeth and hosts.

From: *Endodontics & Dental Traumatology* 1990 February; Volume 6, Number 1, pp. 1-5.

Article Title:
Bacterial invasion into dentinal tubules of human vital and nonvital teeth.

Nagaoka S, Miyazaki Y, Liu HJ, Iwamoto Y, Kitano M, Kawagoe M.

Department of Operative Dentistry and Endodontology, Kagoshima University Dental School, Japan.

ABSTRACT: The difference in resistance to bacterial invasion into the dentinal tubules between vital and nonvital teeth has not been determined. This study was conducted to clarify the effect of vital pulp on bacterial invasion into the dentinal tubules. The specimens were 19 intact pairs of bilateral upper third molars of 19 healthy, young adult male volunteers. In each case, 30 or 150 days before extraction, pulpectomies and root canal fillings were carried out unilaterally and a class V cavity involving the dentin was made on the palatal surface of both the pulpectomized tooth and the nonpulpectomized opposite tooth. The cavities were left unprotected to expose them to oral flora until the extractions were done, and the extracted teeth were examined histologically. When extraction followed 150-day exposure to the oral flora, there was a statistically significant difference in the bacterial invasion rate between the vital and nonvital teeth. It was postulated that vital teeth were much more resistant to bacterial invasion into the dentinal tubules than were nonvital teeth, thereby suggesting that the vital pulp plays some important role in this process.

From: *Journal of Endodontics* 1995 February; Volume 21, Number 2, pp. 70-73.

Article Title:
Bacteremia in conjunction with endodontic therapy.

Debelian GJ, Olsen I, Tronstad L.

Division of Endodontics, Department of Oral Biology, Faculty of Dentistry, University of Oslo, Norway.

ABSTRACT: This study characterizes oral microorganisms believed to have spread from the root canal into the blood stream during and after endodontic therapy of teeth with asymptomatic apical periodontitis. Microbiological samples were taken under aseptic conditions from the root canal of 26 single-rooted teeth in 26 patients. In the endodontic treatment of 13 of the patients (Group 1), the first 3 reamers, sizes 15, 20 and 25, were used to a level 2 mm beyond the apical foramen. In the other 13 patients (Group 2), the instrumentation ended inside the root canal 1 mm short of the apical foramen. Blood samples were taken from the patients during the instrumentation and 10 min after the treatment was completed. Anaerobic microorganisms were isolated from all root canals. In 7 patients of Group 1, *Propionibacterium acnes*, *Peptostreptococcus prevotii*, *Fusobacterium nucleatum*, *Prevotella intermedia* and *Saccharomyces cerevisiae* were recovered from the blood. In 4 patients of Group 2, *P. intermedia*, *Actinomyces israelii*, *Streptococcus intermedius* and *Streptococcus sanguis* were isolated from the blood. Biochemical tests and antibiograms revealed that the isolates from the root canal and blood had identical profiles within the patients, strongly suggesting that the microorganisms isolated from the blood had the root canal as their source.

From: *Endodontics & Dental Traumatology* 1995 June; Volume

11, Number 3, pp. 142-149.

Article Title:
Electrophoresis of whole-cell soluble proteins of microorganisms isolated from bacteremias in endodontic therapy.

Debelian GJ, Olsen I, Tronstad L.

Department of Oral Biology, University of Oslo, Norway.

ABSTRACT: We have previously demonstrated that anaerobic bacteria are the microorganisms most frequently isolated from blood following endodontic therapy of teeth with apical periodontitis. Phenotypic characterisation of the isolates suggested that the bacteria in the blood originated from the root canal. The present experiment using sodium dodecyl sulfate-polyacrylamide gel electrophoresis (SDS-PAGE) was carried out in an effort to verify these findings, and to further study the microorganisms involved in endodontic bacteremias. Soluble cellular proteins were extracted from 11 reference strains and 26 bacterial isolates recovered from the root canal and blood. These included *Propionibacterium acnes*, *Peptostreptococcus prevotii*, *Fusobacterium nucleatum*, *Prevotella intermedia*. *Actinomyces israelii*, *Streptococcus intermedius*, *Streptococcus sanguis*. The electrophoretic patterns mostly confirmed the identity of the isolates as determined by the biochemical and antimicrobial resistance tests. Furthermore, with this typing method the species *Prevotella intermedia* and *Prevotella nigrescens* could be differentiated. These species had been recovered from both root canal and blood. Also, differences between subspecies of *Fusobacterium nucleatum* became evident with SDS-PAGE, and the results indicated that the organism recovered from the root canal and blood was *Fusobacterium nucleatum* subsp. *vincentii*. The electrophoretic patterns of the different organisms isolated from the root canal and the blood were similar, providing further evidence that the bacteria found in the blood originated from the root canal.

From: *European Journal of Oral Sciences* 1996 October-December; Volume 104, Numbers 5-6, pp. 540-546.

Article Title:
Anaerobic bacteremia and fungemia in patients undergoing endodontic therapy: an overview.

Debelian GJ, Olsen I, Tronstad L.

Division of Endodontics, Dental Faculty, University of Oslo, Norway.

ABSTRACT: Oral focal infection, a concept neglected for several decades, is a subject of controversy. Recent progress in classification and identification of oral microorganisms has renewed interest in focal infection. The aim of this study was to use phenotypic and genetic methods to trace microorganisms released into the bloodstream during and after endodontic treatment back to their presumed source—the root canal. Microbiological samples were taken from the root canals of 26 patients with asymptomatic apical periodontitis of single-rooted teeth. The blood of the patients was drawn during and 10 minutes after endodontic therapy. Microorganisms in blood were collected after anaerobic lysis filtration and cultured anaerobically on blood agar plates. The phenotypic methods used for characterization and tracing of microorganisms in blood and root canals were: biochemical and antimicrobial susceptibility test, SDS-PAGE of whole-cell soluble proteins, and gas chromatography of cellular fatty acids. Phenotypic data were verified by DNA restriction patterns and corresponding ribotypes of the root canal and blood isolates by using a computer-assisted system fro gel analysis. All root canals contained anaerobic bacteria. The frequency of bacteremia varied from 31% to 54%. The microorganisms from the root canal and blood presented identical phenotype and genetic characteristics within the patients examined. These characteristics differed between patients. The present study demonstrated that endodontic treatment can be the cause of anaerobic bacteremia and fungemia. The phenotypic and genetic methods used appeared valuable for tracing microorganisms in the blood back to their origin.

From: *Annals of Periodontology* 1998 July; Volume 3, Number 1, pp. 281-287.

Article Title:
The endodontic microflora revisited.

Drucker DB, Lilley JD, Tucker D, Gibbs AC.

Department of Cell and Structural Biology, Turner Dental School, University of Manchester, Great Britain.

ABSTRACT: The microbial flora of 35 dental root canals were examined, taking care to maintain the viability of obligate anaerobes which accounted for 45% of total isolations, while streptococcal species accounted for 24% of the total species isolated. Individual root canals yielded a maximum of eight bacterial species. A total of 40 different species was isolated of which the most prevalent were the facultative anaerobe *Streptococcus sanguis* and the obligate anaerobe, *Peptostreptococcus micros* (both in 23% of root canals), followed by *Eubacterium aerofaciens* and the '*Streptococcus milleri* group' (both 17%) then *Prevotella melaninogenica* (formerly *Bacteroides melaninogenicus*), *Enterococcus faecalis* and *Prevotella oralis* (formerly *Bacteroides oralis*), which were each isolated from 14% of root canals. Highly significant associations were discovered between four pairs of species, viz *P.*

melaninogenica with *P. micros*, *P. melaninogenica* with *P. oralis*, *Prevotella corporis* with *Streptococcus morbillorum* and *Actinomyces odontolyticus* with *E. faecalis*.

From: *Microbios* 1992; Volume 71, Numbers 288-289, pp. 225-234.

Article Title:
Anaerobic flora in endodontic infections.

Chaudhry R, Kalra N, Talwar V, Thakur R.

Department of Microbiology, University College of Medical Sciences, Delhi.

ABSTRACT: Microbiological and clinical data from 56 patients with endodontic infections were evaluated. Samples were collected using autoclaved paper points. Specimens were processed for isolation of aerobic and anaerobic bacteria. Antimicrobial sensitivity and resistance profiles of the recovered isolates were also performed. Forty-nine positive cultures (87.5%) were obtained from the 56 consecutive necrotic root canal systems, which were sampled. A total of 69 aerobic bacteria and 21 anaerobic bacteria were recovered. Aerobic bacteria were isolated from 35 patients (72%), anaerobic bacteria from 3 (6%) and mixed aerobic and anaerobic bacteria from 11 patients (22%). The most common aerobic isolate was *Klebsiella pneumoniae*. The predominant anaerobic isolate was *Bacteroides* species. One isolate was recovered from 25 patients (51%) whereas in the remaining 24 patients (49%) more than 1 isolate were recovered. These data illustrate the polymicrobial nature of endodontic infections in half the patients studied and the role of anaerobic bacteria in a quarter of them.

From: *The Indian Journal of Medical Research* 1997 June; Volume 105, pp. 262-265.

Article Title:
Bacteria in the apical 5 mm of infected root canals.

Baumgartner JC, Falkler WA Jr.

Microbiology Branch, United States Army Institute of Dental Research, Walter Reed Army Medical Center, Washington, DC.

ABSTRACT: Ten freshly extracted teeth, which had carious pulpal exposures and periapical lesions contiguous with the root apex, were placed inside an anaerobic chamber and the apical 5 mm of the root canals cultured. In addition to anaerobic incubation, duplicate cultures were incubated aerobically. Fifty strains of bacteria from the 10 root canals were isolated and identified. The most prominent bacteria cultured from the 10 root canals were *Actinomyces*, *Lactobacillus*, black-pigmented *Bacteroides*, *Peptostreptococcus*, nonpigmented *Bacteroides*, *Veillonella*, *Enterococcus faecalis*, *Fusobacterium nucleatum*, and *Streptococcus mutans*. Of the 50 bacterial isolates, 34 (68%) were strict anaerobes. This study demonstrates the presence of predominantly anaerobic bacteria in the apical 5 mm of infected root canals in teeth with carious pulpal exposures and periapical lesions.

From: *Journal of Endodontics* 1991 August; Volume 17, Number 8, pp. 380-383.

Article Title:
Serious complications of endodontic infections: some cautionary tales.

Walsh LJ.

Department of Dentistry, University of Queensland Dental School.

ABSTRACT: While endodontic (dentoalveolar) abscesses can cause significant morbidity, in susceptible individuals they can pose life-threatening problems. This paper provides an overview of the more serious sequelae of endodontic abscesses, and provides examples of 'high risk' situations in practice in which these serious complications are more likely to occur.

From: *Australian Dental Journal* 1997 June; Volume 42, Number 3, pp. 156-159.

Article Title:
Dentine tubule infection and endodontic therapy implications.

Oguntebi BR.

Department of Endodontics, University of Florida, College of Dentistry, Gainesville 32610-0436.

ABSTRACT: A critical review of the literature suggests that the microenvironment of dentinal tubules appears to favour the selection of relatively few bacterial types irrespective of the aetiology of the infection process; coronal dental caries or pulpar necrosis. These bacteria may constitute an important reservoir from which root canal infection and reinfection may occur following pulp necrosis or during and after endodontic treatment. Previous studies of this microflora have utilized microbiological culture techniques, which need to be supplemented by those that allow in situ demonstration as well as identification of the bacteria. Newer treatment strategies that are designed to eliminate this microflora must include agents that can penetrate the dentinal tubules and destroy these microorganisms, since they are located in an area beyond the host defence mechanisms where they cannot be reached by systemically administered antimicrobial agents.

From: *International Endodontic Journal* 1994 July; Volume 27, Number 4, pp. 218-222.

Article Title:
Implant failures associated with asymptomatic endodontically treated teeth.

Brisman DL, Brisman AS, Moses MS.

Adult Dental Department, Bellevue Hospital Medical Center, New York City, USA.

ABSTRACT: Endosseous root-formed implants occasionally fail to osseointegrate. Causes of failure include infection, overheating of the bone, habitual smoking, systemic disease, transmucosal overloading, excessive surgical trauma and implant placement adjacent to teeth demonstrating periapical pathology. CASE DESCRIPTION: In this article, the authors present another possible cause of implant failure. The cases of four patients who received endosseous root-formed implants are discussed. Each patient demonstrated signs of infection after initial implant placement. The common factor in each failing implant was its placement adjacent to an asymptomatic endodontically treated tooth with no clinical or radiographic evidence of pathology. CLINICAL IMPLICATIONS: These patients demonstrate the importance of evaluating and possibly retreating or extracting adjacent endodontically treated teeth before placing implants.

From: *The Journal of the American Dental Association* 2001 February; Volume 132, Number 2, 191-195.

APPENDIX III

CAUSES OF CAVITATIONS AND ASSOCIATED CONDITIONS

Overview of Causes

Cavitational disease, or ischemic osteonecrosis, results from both systemic and local problems at a number of sites in the body.

Ischemic osteonecrosis is not so much a disease in its own right as it is the localized result of anything which significantly reduces the blood flow through the bone marrow. Ischemic osteonecrosis of the head of the femur was once called "coronary disease of the hip" because of the associated marrow ischemia (reduced blood flow) and infarction (complete blockage of a vessel).

Overview of Causes (cont.)

In cases of ischemic osteonecrosis involving the femoral head, the list of diseases and biological phenomena capable of producing this damage has grown to an impressive size during recent years. Some of these etiologic factors are much more significant than others. Some factors are primary causes and other factors act as triggering mechanisms or "second hits" in persons otherwise susceptible to bone marrow blood flow problems.

Jaws are especially susceptible to cavitations and ischemic osteonecrosis for several reasons.

The jaws are especially susceptible to reduced blood flow problems. Trauma and infection are the primary triggering events for osteonecrosis and no other bones come close to the level of trauma and infection experienced by the jaws, e.g. tooth and gum infections, tooth extractions, trauma (a fist to the face, perhaps?), and oral or root canal (endodontic) or gum (periodontic) surgery. To these potential causes we can add others which are rather unique to dental procedures: local anesthetics used to numb to jaw for tooth procedures or oral surgery contain powerful chemicals (vasoconstrictors, e.g. epinephrine) designed to drastically reduce the blood flow in the area, thereby keeping the anesthetic in place longer and allowing more time to work. This is wonderful for the procedure itself but can be disastrous for someone with any one of the undiagnosed hypercoagulation disorders to be mentioned. Moreover, the poor outflow characteristic of

Overview of Causes (cont.)	osteonecrosis means that the vasoconstrictor can remain in the area much, much longer than the few minutes needed for profound local anesthesia. And to add injury to insult, literally, the reperfusion of the bone after the vasoconstrictor wears off releases large numbers of tissue-damaging reactive oxygen species. Normal tissues can withstand this onslaught nicely, but a nutrient-starved ischemic marrow does not maintain its marginal health status as well.
Hypercoagulation States	Hypercoagulation (a state where the blood clots more readily) is common. The most important underlying, and almost always undiagnosed, susceptibility to cavitations comes from coagulation disorders, i.e., a Ask about family history of clotting problems. This hypercoagulation problem might be suggested by a family history of stroke and heart attacks at an early age (less than 55 years), hip replacement or "arthritis" (especially at an early age), and deep vein thrombosis. Hypercoagulation may be a life-threatening problem. Always keep in mind that the presence of a hypercoagulation state makes the patient susceptible to stroke, myocardial infarction, deep vein thrombosis, and other serious or life-threatening conditions. Usually a secondary problem or "triggering event" must occur, such as local infection, trauma, medications, etc.

Hypercoagulation States (cont.)	**There are other diseases associated with hypercoagulation. A number of diseases/factors have been associated with hypercoagulation states, including:** - Behçet's disease - Chronic fatigue syndrome - Fibromyalgia - Irritable bowel syndrome - Sickle cell crisis - Migraine headaches The significance of these associations is not yet known, but these disorders appear to occur frequently in patients with ischemic osteonecrosis (no formal investigation has yet been done to prove this).
Hormones	Estrogen replacement therapy can be a cause. Estrogen enhances coagulation. In persons with a hypercoagulation state (at least 6% of the population) the risk of thrombosis from estrogen use increases, sometimes dramatically. For example, the risk for a person with a single hypercoagulation disorder of forming a clot somewhere in the body (not just the jaws) is increased by more than 80 times when estrogen replacement is given. The orthopedic literature sometimes refers to estrogen-related ischemic osteonecrosis.

Hormones (cont.)

Pregnancy is associated with increased estrogen levels. Because of this, pregnant women are at an elevated risk of developing ischemic osteonecrosis, especially of the hip. A mild, self-limiting condition that is a precursor to osteonecrosis, transient ischemic osteoporosis, often spontaneously regresses with immobility after the birth of the child. Multiple joints may be involved, sometimes moving from one to another over time (migratory ischemic osteoporosis).

Hypercortisolism (excess corticosteroid presence) is another cause of osteonecrosis. It can result from either natural production or from the common practice of prescribing prednisone or prednisolone to prevent swelling after oral surgical procedures. Corticosteroid use is the most common cause of non-traumatic osteonecrosis. Although the risk appears to be dose-dependent and time-of-use dependent, there are reports of massive hip disease from a single week's use of Medrol. The orthopedic literature contains articles pertaining to corticosteroid-induced osteonecrosis. The mechanism is unclear.

Hypothyroidism. Low levels of thyroid hormone have been associated with an increased risk of developing ischemic osteonecrosis of the hip, probably because the diminished metabolism produced by this condition reduces blood flow rates throughout the body.

Autoimmunity and Hypersensitivity	Systemic lupus erythematosus. Antiphospholipid syndrome
Miscellaneous Factors	Other causes.

Recurring maxillary sinus infections with the potential seeding of bacteria in the alveolar bone, producing osteomyelitis (bone infection), is a major risk factor. The inflammatory mediators at work in this chronic process are capable of increasing local and systemic coagulation. This is generally not a problem for a normal person but can be, again, disastrous for the 6% or more of us who have undiagnosed or "silent" hypercoagulation states.

Gaucher's disease.

This lipid storage disease is associated with hyperviscosity, thrombocytopenia, and decreased factor IX and protein C. It has been suggested that when the very large lesional cells, Gaucher cells, enter the blood vessels they act as emboli and when they fragment their breakdown products they trigger excess intravascular coagulation, leading to thrombosis and hemorrhage (microinfarctions). Just before a crisis, there is radioisotopic evidence of ischemia, but it may be days or several months after the acute pain onset before a biopsy will show obvious osteonecrosis

Diseases and conditions associated with osteonecrosis (any bone).

Disease or Etiologic Factor	Subcategories
Alcohol Abuse	Cirrhosis
	Pancreatitis
Arthritis	Subchondral cyst
	Subchondral marrow edema
Atmospheric Pressure Variations	Caisson's disease
	Deep sea diving
Blood dyscrasias	Disseminated intravascular coagulation (DIC)
	Sickle cell anemia
Cancer	Leukemia
	Chemotherapy for cancer
	Cancer-induced hypercoagulation
	Lymphoma
	Metastatic intraosseous carcinoma
	Radiation therapy for cancer
Chronic Inactivity	Bedridden
	Full body cast
	Paraplegic
Corticosteriods	Hypercortisolism
	Inflammatory bowel disease
	Lupus erythematosus
	Transplants
Estrogen	Birth control pills
	Estrogen replacement therapy
	Fertility drugs
	Pregnancy
	Prostate chemotherapy
	Transient ischemic osteoporosis

Disease or Etiologic Factor	Subcategories
Hypercoagulable state, local	Acute infection/inflammation Chronic infection/inflammation Increased intramedullary pressures
Hypercoagulable state, systemic	Antiphospholipid antibody syndrome Factor V Leiden gene mutation Hyperhomocysteinemia Homozygosity for MTHFR* or CBS * Protein C deficiency Protein S deficiency
Hyperlipidemia & embolic fat	Diabetes mellitus Dysbaric phenomena Fracture of bone Hemoglobinopathies Osteomyelitis, acute
Hypersensitivity reactions	Allograft organ rejection Anaphylactic shock Immune globulin therapy Shwartzman reaction to endotoxin Transfusion reactions
Hypertension	
Hypothyroidism	
Incomplete removal of the periodontal ligament at the time of tooth extraction	
Inflammation, intraosseous	
Inflammation, intraosseous	Infection, bacterial and viral Trauma (mild or severe) Autoimmunity/ hypersensitivity

Disease or Etiologic Factor	Subcategories
Neuro-damage	Brain injury/surgery
Osteoporosis	Regional or generalized
Starvation	Anorexia nervosa
Storage diseases	Gaucher's disease
Tobacco use	Tobacco smoking
Vascular occlusive disease	Atherosclerosis
Vasculitis Vasoconstriction	Local anesthesia (with vasoconstrictor)
	Raynaud's phenomenon
	Tobacco use

* MTHFR: methylene tetrahydrofolate reductase; CBS: cystathionine beta-synthetase

The above information has been reproduced, with some modifications, with the permission of Dr. Jerry Bouquot, The Maxillofacial Center, 165 Scott Avenue, Suite 100, Morgantown, WV 26508 USA

Phone: 304-292-4429 Fax: 304-291-5149 Email: MFC@aol.com

Website: www.maxillofacialcenter.com

Appendix IV

Photographs

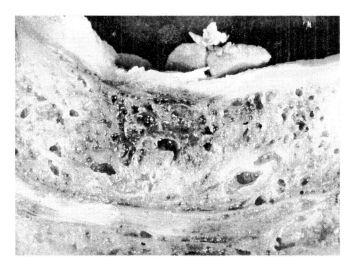

This is a picture of a cadaver mandible (lower jaw) that is split in sagital section (front to back). This person had severe facial pain due to ischemic osteonecrosis/chronic osteomyelitis that involved a large part of the lower jaw including the neurovascular bundle. Any infection or toxin release would have an easy pathway to the rest of the body via the large nerves and blood vessels that pass through this diseased bone.
(Photo courtesy J.E. Bouquot, D.D.S., M.S.D.)

The Roots of Disease

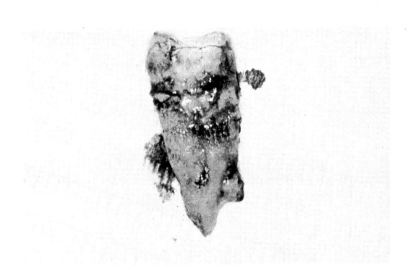

This tooth has an infected granuloma located behind the root rather than at the apex of the root. This lesion would not be visible on a two dimensional dental x-ray. Therefore dentists should never rely on x-rays alone to diagnose the presence of a granuloma or a cyst.

(Photo: Robert Kulacz, D.D.S.)

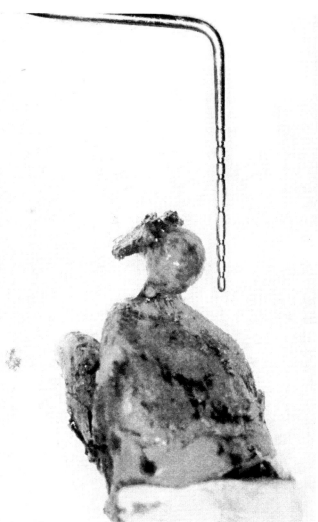

There is a 5mm granuloma at the peri-apical (tip) of the root. This infection had destroyed and infected the bone of the jaw.
(Photo: Robert Kulacz, D.D.S.)

The Roots of Disease

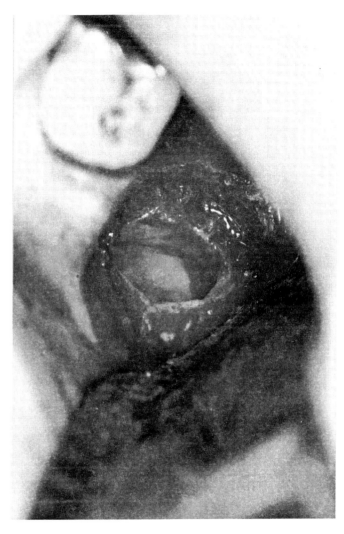

Hole in the maxilla (upper jaw) that extends into the sinus cavity. This opening was caused by extensive infection around the tip of the tooth adjacent to the sinus floor.
(Photo: Robert Kulacz, D.D.S.)

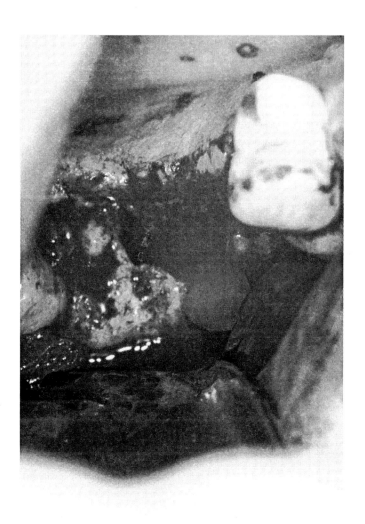

Large opening into the sinus cavity through the maxillary bone following a previous tooth extraction. Treatment required the surgical placement of a barrier membrane made of a resorbable material to close this large bone defect.
(Photo: Robert Kulacz, D.D.S.)

The Roots of Disease

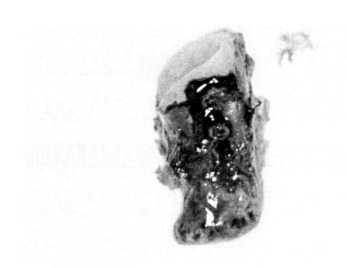

Extracted root canal tooth that gave the patient no clinical symptoms such as pain. There is extensive infected tissue around this tooth. This tooth emitted a strong and pungent odor.
(Photo: Robert Kulacz, D.D.S.)

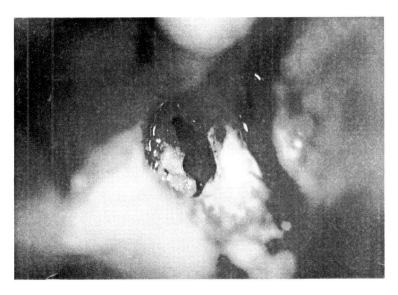

Cavitation at the area of a previously extracted wisdom tooth site. Surgery revealed healed bone over the cavitation as is common in many cases. Exploration into the cavitation revealed a combination of diseased black tissue as well as hollow unhealed bone.

(Photo: Robert Kulacz, D.D.S.)

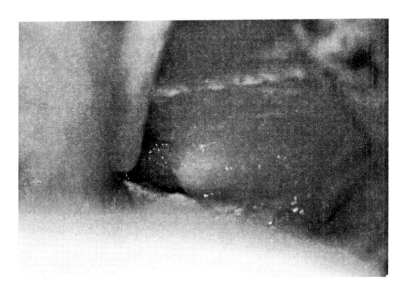

Surgery of the right mandible on a patient with atypical facial pain with referred pain to the right shoulder area. The neurovascular bundle was completely exposed revealing extensive osteonecrotic bone beneath the nerve bundle. This patient experienced a significant and immediate reduction in facial pain and almost total elimination of shoulder pain.
(Photo: Robert Kulacz, D.D.S.)

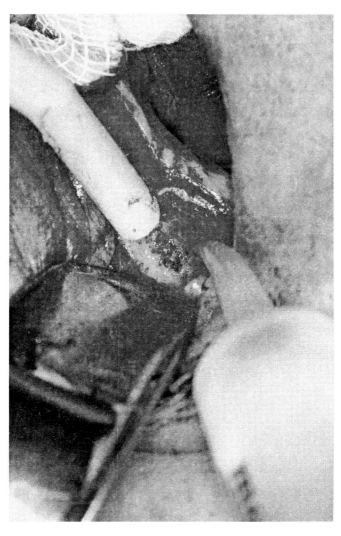

Dark area in the bone is remnants of mercury amalgam that was placed into a tooth during an apicoectomy procedure. The tooth was subsequently extracted yet amalgam remained in the bone. Amalgam extended into the maxillary sinus cavity.
(Photo: Robert Kulacz, D.D.S.)

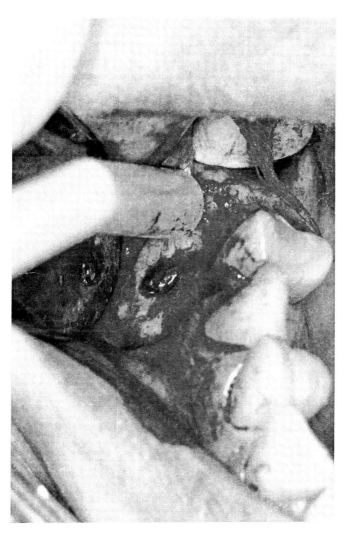

Previous apicoectomy left a hole in the bone with extensive necrotic bone. Mercury amalgam was present in the surrounding jawbone.

(Photo: Robert Kulacz, D.D.S.)

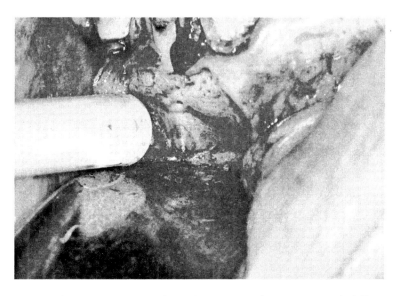

Apex of root canal tooth with gutt-percha root canal filling material extending beyond the tip of the root. Infection and/or the root canal procedure itself caused a perforation in the front plate of jawbone.

(Photo: Robert Kulacz, D.D.S.)

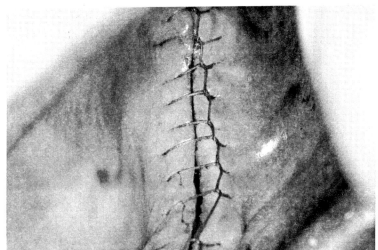

Surgical site closed with a running box lock suture. Primary closure of the surgical site prevents the migration of microorganisms into the site thereby reducing the incidence of re-infection.

(Photo: Robert Kulacz, D.D.S.)

APPENDIX V

RESOURCES

Suggested Readings

Huggins, Hal and Thomas. Levy. (1999) *Uninformed Consent. The Hidden Dangers in Dental Care.* Charlottesville, VA: Hampton Roads Publishing Company, Inc.

Levy, Thomas. (2001) *Optimal Nutrition for Optimal Health. The Real Truth About Eating Right for Weight Loss, Detoxification, Low Cholesterol, Better Digestion, and Overall Well-Being.* New York, NY: Keats Publishing (division of McGraw-Hill).

Meinig, George. (1996) *Root Canal Cover-Up.* Ojai, CA: Bion Publishing.

Huggins, Hal. (1993) *It's All In Your Head. The Link Between Mercury Amalgams and Illness.* Garden City Park, NY: Avery Publishing Group, Inc.

Price, Weston. (1923) *Dental Infection: Oral and Systemic.* Volume 1. Cleveland, OH: The Penton Publishing Company.

Price, Weston. (1923) *Dental Infections and the Degenerative Diseases.* Volume II. Cleveland, OH: The Penton Publishing Company.

Kulish, Peter. (1999) *Conquering Pain. The Art of Healing with Biomagnetism.* Fountainville, PA: Fountainville Press.

Davis, Albert and Walter Rawls. (1975) *The Magnetic Effect.* Kansas City, MO: Acres U.S.A.

Davis, Albert and Walter Rawls. (1979) *The Magnetic Blueprint of Life.* Kansas City, MO: Acres U.S.A.

Hussar, Christopher, DO, DDS and Robert Kulacz, DDS (2002) *Oral Infections: Diagnosis and Treatment.* Xlibris Publishing

Suggested Resources

1. **Regarding dental toxicity, dental infections, and assistance in getting a Total Dental Revision:**

Robert Kulacz, D.D.S.
Office: (914) 288-0993
E-mail: robertkulacz@earthlink.net
Website: www.drkulacz.com

Thomas E. Levy, M.D., J.D.
Office: (719) 548-1600
Toll-free: (800) 331-2303
Fax: (719) 572-8081
E-mail: televymd@yahoo.com
Website: www.TomLevyMD.com

To subscribe to "Health E-Bytes," Dr. Levy's free newsletter, send your email address to the e-mail address above.

Christopher Hussar, D.O., D.D.S.
Office: (775) 826-1200
E-mail: drhussar@hotmail.com
Website: www.drhussar.com

Hal A. Huggins, D.D.S., M.S.

Office: (719) 522-0566
Toll-free: (866) 948-4638
Fax: (719) 548-8220
Website: www.hugnet.com

Occidental Institute Research Foundation: non-profit research organization for practitioners of biological medicine. An information and technology bridge between Germany and English speaking doctors. Not for patient referrals.
Website: www.oirf.com
Telephone: (250) 497-6020

2. **Regarding serum biocompatibility testing for replacement dental materials:**

Peak Energy Performance, Inc.
Use contact information given above for Dr. Levy
Website: www.PeakEnergy.com

3. **Books by Dr. Weston Price and related information:**

Price-Pottenger Nutrition Foundation
Office: (619) 574-7763
Toll-free: (800) 366-3748
Fax: (619) 574-1314
E-mail: info@price-pottenger.org
Website: www.price-pottenger.org

4. **For more information on obtaining and using bio-magnets:**

Magnetizer
Office: (215) 249-1200
Fax: (215) 249-3161
E-mail: mgimag@magnetizer.com
Website: www.magnetizer.com

APPENDIX VI

ABOUT THE AUTHORS

Robert Kulacz, D.D.S.
Dr. Kulacz attended The University of California at San Diego and graduated from The State University of New York at Cortland with a degree in biology and a minor in chemistry in 1982. He attended New York University College of Dentistry where he received his dental degree in 1986. Dr. Kulacz did a post-graduate training program sponsored by Brookdale Hospital in Brooklyn, N.Y. in dental implant surgery and implant restoration in 1989. He was an instructor in the department of human anatomy at NYU College of Dentistry in 1992.

Dr. Kulacz abandoned his traditional dental practice in 1997 after learning of the dangers of the dental procedures he was performing and currently limits his practice to oral surgery, treating cavitations and other oral infections.

The Roots of Disease is his first book but will certainly not be his last. He intends to divide his time between clinical practice, research, and writing.

In addition to caring for his four-year-old twin daughters, and sharing his life with his physician wife Susan, Dr. Kulacz is an accomplished pilot and musician, and is currently training for an Ironman triathlon. Dr. Kulacz lives and practices in Westchester County, New York.

Thomas E. Levy, M.D., J.D.

Dr. Levy received his undergraduate degree in biology from the Johns Hopkins University in 1972. He then received his medical degree from Tulane Medical School in 1976. He specialized in the fields of internal medicine and cardiology, receiving board certification in internal medicine in 1979 and subspecialty board certification in cardiology in 1981. Dr. Levy served as an assistant professor of medicine at Tulane Medical School from 1981 to 1983. Since 1999, Dr. Levy has also been an assistant professor at the Capital University of Integrative Medicine in Washington, D.C.

In 1998 Dr. Levy received his law degree from the University of Denver. He has been admitted to the bars of both the state of Colorado and the District of Columbia. He became a Diplomate of the American College of Forensic Examiners in 1999.

Dr. Levy is also an established medical author. In 1999, he co-authored *Uninformed Consent: The Hidden Dangers in Dental Care* with Dr. Hal Huggins. In 2001 he also wrote *Optimal Nutrition for Optimal Health*. Dr. Levy is presently working on a series of books about the documented yet little known facts about the many benefits of properly dosed vitamin C. He also writes a periodic email newsletter, "Health E-Bytes."

BVG